Table of Contents

Introduction

Emergency department nurses work with patients of all ages, and face many challenges in this specialty area. They may have little or no information about the patient, who may be unconscious and unaccompanied by a family member who can provide information. For these reasons, a rapid physical assessment may provide the only data that can be used for immediate emergency treatment. It may not even be possible to get an informed consent in this environment.

Patient's needs are often highly specialized so the emergency nurse must be flexible and fully knowledgeable. Ailments ranging from ectopic pregnancies to suicide attempts to blast injuries to ocular emergencies will present in the ER - they represent specialty needs, such as obstetrics, mental health, trauma and ophthalmology, respectively, and the emergency nurse must competently employ specialized skills in all of these disciplines.

Nurses also must be able to use many different types of equipment and technology, and have the expertise necessary for sound critical thinking, professional judgment, communication, and collaboration skills.

Assessment and treatment must be accurate and timely. These patients are typically in a life-threatening condition. When not in a life-threatening condition, the workflow of the area must be maintained by fast tracking those who have a minor condition so they can be discharge to the home after treatment and discharge teaching. For example, a child with a fractured arm or with a sore throat may be fast tracked and treated, which may include following up with a specialist or their family practitioner, so they can be sent back to their home and activities of daily living.

Emergency nurses work in collaboration with other multidisciplinary members of the emergency care department. They coordinate and collaborate with medical doctors, within the emergency area and those with other specialized practices, such as ophthalmology or gynecology. They also work side by side with respiratory therapists, nurse practitioners, clinical nurse specialists, pharmacists, radiology staff, laboratory staff, social workers, dieticians, paramedics from the community and law enforcement officers, when the patient is accused of a crime.

Section 1: Treating Emergencies

Cardiovascular Emergencies

Acute Coronary Syndrome (ACS)

Any condition brought on by the sudden reduction of blood flow to the heart is considered a life-threatening condition, known as acute coronary syndrome (ACS).

Signs and Symptoms

ACS mimics a heart attack. The signs and symptoms include diaphoresis, dyspnea, nausea and vomiting, angina, chest pain and referred pain.

Treatment

Depending on the symptoms and the extent of the artery blockage, medications and/or surgery may be necessary. Medications include aspirin, thrombolytic drugs, nitroglycerin, angiotensin-converting enzymes, ACE inhibitors, angiotensin receptor blockers, beta-blockers, calcium channel blockers, cholesterol-lowering drugs, and anticoagulants.

When medications do not adequately restore cardiac function, surgical procedures, such as angioplasty and a stent, or coronary bypass surgery, may be necessary.

Aneurysm/Dissection

An aneurysm is a balloon-like bulge in an artery. Certain medical problems, genetic conditions or trauma can damage arterial walls, and the force of the blood pushing against these weakened or injured walls can lead to the formation of an aneurysm.

An aneurysm can grow quite large and rupture and/or dissect without any symptomatic warning, thus causing a massive life-threatening hemorrhage, unless it is immediately diagnosed and treated. A split in one or more of the artery walls, which is known as a dissection, causes bleeding into and along the layers of the artery wall.

Ruptures and dissection are often fatal.

Signs and Symptoms

The signs and symptoms vary depending on the type and location of the aneurysm, and whether it has ruptured and/or affected the body's blood flow. Most aneurysms are asymptomatic, and develop slowly and silently over years until a rupture occurs.

Abdominal aortic aneurysms tend to develop slowly, but initial symptoms include a throbbing in the abdomen, a deep pain in the back or side of the abdomen, and a steady pain in the abdomen that lasts for hours or days. Once the rupture occurs, symptoms such as nausea, vomiting, constipation, problems urinating, clammy skin, lightheadedness, a rapid pulse and the signs and symptoms of hypovolemic shock occur.

Thoracic aortic aneurysms may also not present symptoms until it dissects or grows large enough to lead to symptoms, such as jaw, neck, back or chest pain, coughing and/or hoarseness, shortness of breath, dyspnea and difficulty swallowing. Sudden, severe, sharp or stabbing pain can start in the back and move to the abdomen, if the aneurysm ruptures or dissects. Pain may present in the chest and arms, and then shock can occur quickly. Left untreated, organ damage or death can occur.

Treatment

Treatment for aneurysms includes antihypertensive medications, such as beta-blockers or calcium channel blockers, which lower blood pressure and relax the blood vessels, both of which can prevent a rupture.

Another treatment option is surgery. This is usually recommended if the aneurysm is growing quickly or the patient is at risk of rupture or dissection. The main types of surgery include open abdominal (or open chest) repair and endovascular repair.

Cardiopulmonary Arrest

Cardiopulmonary arrest is defined as an unexpected and sudden loss of cardiac function, the cessation of breathing and the loss of consciousness. This is due to an electrical disturbance in the heart, which disrupts its pumping action and stops the flow of blood to rest of the body.

Signs and Symptoms

The signs and symptoms that accompany sudden cardiac arrest occur immediately and dramatically. These signs and symptoms include loss of consciousness, lack of breathing and pulse, and collapse.

Usually there is no warning or symptoms prior to a sudden cardiac arrest, but in some cases, weakness, shortness of breath, fainting, fatigue, chest pain, dizziness, blackouts, palpitations and vomiting may occur.

Treatment

The immediate treatment for sudden cardiac arrest is CPR. Advanced care for ventricular fibrillation includes defibrillation. Other treatments include the following:

- Medications, such as anti-arrhythmic drugs for treatment of arrhythmias, beta-blockers, angiotensin-converting enzyme (ACE) inhibitors, calcium channel blockers or amiodarone
- Implantable cardioverter-defibrillator (ICD)
- Coronary bypass surgery
- Coronary angioplasty
- Corrective heart surgery
- Radiofrequency catheter ablation
- Heart transplant

Normal Cardiac Rhythms and Dysrhythmias

Normal Sinus Rhythm

Normal sinus rhythm is the normal rhythm of the heart that comes from the heart's natural pacemaker, which is the SA node. The rate of the normal sinus rhythm is between 60 and 100 beats per minute; a P wave occurs before each QRS complex, the QRS complex is from 0.04–0.11 seconds, and the PR intervals are normal and from 0.12–0.20 seconds. All other cardiac rhythms are considered dysrhythmias and not normal.

Sinus Bradycardia and Sinus Tachycardia

Bradycardia is a rate less than 60 beats per minute; tachycardia is a rate of more than 100 beats per minute. Both of these rhythms have all the features of a normal sinus rhythm with the exception of the rate.

Sinus bradycardia occurs when the SA node takes longer than normal to depolarize due to some vagal, parasympathetic stimulation. This dysrhythmia extends the duration of diastole and reduces cardiac output. It occurs primarily among those with coronary artery disease, upon vagal stimulation, during a myocardial infarction, secondary to increased intracranial pressure, as a side effect of medications, such as beta-blockers and digitalis, and during sleep. Healthy athletes may also present with sinus bradycardia.

Sinus tachycardia occurs when the SA node depolarizes more quickly than normal. This dysrhythmia reduces cardiac output and coronary artery perfusion. The duration of diastole is shorter than normal sinus rhythm. Sinus tachycardia is associated with caffeine use, pain, hyperthyroidism, sympathetic nervous system stimulation, stress, exercise, and a cardiovascular response to hypovolemia and hypotension.

Sinus Arrhythmia

Sinus arrhythmia is present when there are cyclical vagal variations in the sinus rhythm. This abnormal (but not life-threatening) rhythm speeds the SA node up at the end of respiratory inspiration and slows it down at the end of respiratory expiration. This dysrhythmia occurs primarily among otherwise healthy children and young adults.

Premature Atrial Contractions

Premature atrial contractions (PACs or APCs) occur as the result of irritable atrial cells, rather than the SA node. A normal QRS complex occurs, but it is preceded by a premature and early occurring P wave. This dysrhythmia is associated with a number of risk factors, including nicotine use, fatigue, alcohol, digitalis, electrolyte imbalances, ischemia and hypoxia.

Atrial Flutter

Atrial flutter occurs when the AV node blocks rapid atrial depolarization rates of about 300 beats per minute. It can be irregular or regular. The danger of thrombosis is present but less than with atrial fibrillation.

Heart failure, chronic pulmonary disease and right-sided heart enlargement can cause atrial flutter. This cardiac arrhythmia is treated with amiodarone, digitalis, calcium channel blockers, beta-blockers, and cardioversion, when indicated.

Paroxysmal Supraventricular Tachycardia

This arrhythmia is caused by the takeover of the SA node pacemaker function by the atria or AV junction. It often appears and disappears in a rapid manner and is typically self-limiting.

Some of the causes of paroxysmal supraventricular tachycardia are stress, nicotine, electrolyte imbalance, caffeine, alcohol, hypoxic episodes and ischemia. This cardiac arrhythmia can often be resolved with simple coughing or carotid massage. Other treatment options include intravenous adenosine and cardioversion if the patient remains unstable after other treatments.

Asystole

Asystole, also known as a flat line, is the complete absence of and cessation of all ventricular activity, despite the fact that atrial impulses and P waves may appear on the ECG.

Immediate advanced life support is necessary. Intravenous adrenaline, sodium bicarbonate and atropine, as well as 100% oxygen, are given in hopes of preserving life.

Atrial Fibrillation

Atrial fibrillation is a relatively common arrhythmia, especially among the elderly and those patients with mitral valve disorders, pulmonary embolus, hypoxia and congestive heart disease.

Cardiac output is decreased and, at times, emergency treatment for severely affected patients includes cardioversion. Anticoagulation heparin or low molecular weight heparin is administered prior to cardioversion to prevent thromboembolism. The long-term management of atrial fibrillation includes warfarin, aspirin, cardiac rate and rhythm controlling medications, as well as newer medications such as rivaroxaban and dabigatran.

First-Degree Atrioventricular Block

First-degree atrioventricular block is usually asymptomatic. It occurs due to a delay in the AV node impulse that prolongs the PR interval. The P wave is present before each QRS complex.

This heart block can occur prior to a more severe form of heart block. Treatment is not indicated unless the patient is symptomatic.

Second-Degree Atrioventricular Block, Type I

Second-degree atrioventricular (AV) block type I, also referred to as Mobitz type 1/Wenckebach, occurs when there are progressive conduction delays through the AV node. These delays progressively lengthen the PR interval until a missing QRS interval and a non-conducted P wave occur.

Treatment is usually not indicated unless it becomes symptomatic. Digoxin sometimes causes this dysrhythmia.

Second-Degree Atrioventricular Block, Type II

Second-degree AV block type II, also referred to as Mobitz type 2, occurs when the AV node impulses are blocked as they attempt to reach the ventricles. This arrhythmia can lead to a complete heart block. Treatment includes a temporary pacemaker, supplemental oxygen and intravenous atropine.

Complete Heart Block (Third Degree Heart Block)

Third-degree heart block, also called complete AV disassociation, occurs when there are no atrial impulses to the ventricle. Because of this, a ventricular or junctional pacemaker takes over, thus causing a lack of coordination between the atria and ventricles. The ventricular and atrial cardiac rates differ and the QRS complex is wide when the impulse comes from the ventricle.

Complete heart block can be caused by a variety of medications, such as beta-blockers and digoxin. It is commonly associated with acute rheumatic fever, coronary heart disease, myocardial infarction and atrial septal defects.

Some of the signs and symptoms can include syncope, an altered level of consciousness, and chest pain. Emergency treatment, when necessary, includes immediate cardiac pacing and preparation for emergency basic and advanced life support to prevent cardiac arrest.

Premature Ventricular Contractions

Premature ventricular contractions, or premature ventricular complexes, premature ventricular ectopic beats and extrasystole, are life threatening. They occur when ventricular irritability causes abnormal impulses from an ectopic area in the ventricle. A number of factors cause them, including ischemia, electrolyte imbalances, hypoxia, acidosis, and digitalis toxicity.

Premature ventricular contractions can occur in isolation, as a single focus, or in clusters (multifocal). For example, a multifocal pattern can occur every other heartbeat, or every third heartbeat. These multifocal patterns are called bigeminy and trigeminy, respectively; a couplet is two PVCs in succession and a triplet is three PVCs in succession.

Ventricular Tachycardia

With ventricular tachycardia, all cardiac impulses come from the ventricle rather than the atrium. This arrhythmia is extremely dangerous and often leads to ventricular fibrillation and asystole, unless treated immediately and effectively. These ventricular impulses widen the QRS complex and the cardiac rate becomes dangerously rapid and highly inefficient; therefore, profound hemodynamic compromise and instability can occur very quickly.

Dizziness and decreased level of consciousness are highly indicative of ventricular tachycardia. Emergency interventions include cardioversion, intravenous lidocaine and magnesium sulfate, and antiarrhythmic medications such as amiodarone.

Ventricular Fibrillation

Ventricular fibrillation is characterized by chaotic and rapid signals from ectopic ventricular sites. It is accompanied by <u>no</u> cardiac output because all cardiac contractions are ineffective. Death will occur if this rhythm persists for more than six minutes.

The treatment involves immediate advanced life support, including defibrillation, intravenous adrenaline and 100% supplemental oxygen. A lack of treatment leads to asystole.

Endocarditis

Endocarditis is an inflammation and infection of the endocardium or the inner lining of the heart. It is most often associated with an artificial heart or a number of different heart defects.

Signs and Symptoms

Endocarditis can affect different people in different ways. Some of the common signs and symptoms include:

- Chills
- Fever
- Night sweats
- Fatigue
- Shortness of breath
- Body aches
- Paleness
- Swelling in the feet, legs or abdomen
- Gross or occult hematuria
- Tenderness of the spleen
- Osler's nodes, which are red, tender spots that can be seen under the skin of the fingers

Some of the complications of endocarditis include a cerebrovascular accident, organ damage, heart failure, and infections that can spread to other parts of the body.

Treatment

The treatment of endocarditis begins with antibiotics; if the heart valve is damaged, surgery may be required.

Heart Failure

In the past, heart failure was referred to as congestive cardiac failure (CCF). The population at greatest risk for heart failure is the elderly; this increases as the patient advances in age.

Heart failure, simply defined, is a failure of the heart's ability to pump sufficient oxygenated blood to meet the demands and requirements of the body's tissues. Some of the most common causes of heart failure include hypertension, ischemic heart disease, and cardiomyopathy. Left ventricular systolic compromise is the most common underlying cause of heart failure, but right-sided ventricular dysfunction as well as biventricular failure are also causes.

Left ventricular failure is most commonly caused by:

- Systemic hypertension
- Cardiomyopathy
- Bacterial endocarditis
- Myocardial infarction
- Aortic stenosis
- Aortic regurgitation
- Mitral regurgitation

Right ventricular failure is most often associated with mitral stenosis, pulmonary hypertension, bacterial endocarditis, and right ventricular infarction.

Biventricular heart failure is typically the result of cardiomyopathy, myocarditis, left ventricular failure, dysrhythmias, anemia, and thyrotoxicosis.

Signs and Symptoms

Poor heart contractions manifest in terms of a number of signs and symptoms including fluid retention, dyspnea, tachycardia, fatigue, pallor, hypotension, lethargy, activity intolerance and anxiety.

Pathophysiologically, renal, hemodynamic, neural, and hormonal changes can also occur due to heart failure.

Heart failure is treated with a number of different drugs, including diuretics to reduce fluid overload, ACE inhibitors, angiotensin II receptor antagonists (when the patient cannot tolerate ACE inhibitors), and beta-blockers. Treatment can also include biventricular pacing, an implanted cardioverter defibrillator, restricted fluid intake, a low-sodium diet and a medically approved exercise routine.

Hypertension and Hypertensive Crisis

Hypertension, or high blood pressure, is a serious condition that can result in coronary heart disease, heart failure, stroke, kidney failure, and a wide variety of other health problems, including death.

Hypertensive crisis is a rapid, sudden and significant rise in blood pressure that typically evolves for a couple of hours without warning; it is a life threatening disorder; therefore, immediate intervention within two hours is necessary to prevent widespread organ damage.

Signs and Symptoms

Hypertensive crisis presents with a diastolic blood pressure above 120 mmHg and central nervous system compromise. The signs and symptoms can include an altered level of consciousness, headache, cardiovascular compromise, chest pain, angina, myocardial infarction, heart failure, hematuria, oliguria, renal compromise, and renal failure.

Treatment

Emergency intravenous medications for hypertensive crisis include vasodilators like sodium nitroprusside, which dilates both the arteries and the veins, as well as reducing preload and after load with a minimal effect on cardiac output. Beta-blockers and ACE inhibitors are also effective. These emergency intravenous medications should decrease blood pressure by approximately 30% within half an hour.

Nursing interventions include monitoring the patient's blood pressure, preventing complications, assessing the central nervous system and cardiovascular system and continuous monitoring of the patient's status.

Less dramatic cases of hypertension can be treated with lifestyle changes, such as eating a healthy diet, staying physically active, maintaining a healthy weight, quitting smoking, practicing stress management and taking prescribed medications, which include:

- Diuretics
- Beta blockers
- ACE inhibitors
- Angiotensin II receptor blockers
- Calcium channel blockers
- Alpha-blockers
- Alpha-beta blockers
- Nervous system inhibitors
- Vasodilators

Pericardial/Cardiac Tamponade

Pericardial tamponade, also known as cardiac tamponade, occurs when a fluid (often but not always blood) fills the sac between the heart and the heart muscles. This collection of fluid results in pressure around the heart, preventing the heart's ventricles from expanding fully and interfering with normal cardiac function.

Signs and Symptoms

Signs and symptoms include fainting, dizziness, loss of consciousness, rapid breathing, anxiety, restlessness, low blood pressure, weakness, breathing troubles, and discomfort that can only be relieved by sitting forward or leaning forward.

Treatment

Once the patient is stabilized, pericardiocentesis or thoracotomy should be performed. In some cases, a portion of the pericardium may have to be surgically removed in order to help relieve the pressure on the patient's heart. Oxygen, fluids and medications to increase the patient's blood pressure should also be given.

Pericarditis

Pericarditis is an acute inflammation and irritation of the pericardium, which is the two-layered sac containing serous fluid surrounding the myocardium of the heart. Pericarditis is more common among males than females. A major complication of pericarditis is cardiac tamponade.

Some of the risk factors associated with pericarditis include infection, a malignancy (breast cancer, lung cancer, melanoma and lymphoma), radiation therapy, connective tissue diseases, such as scleroderma, systemic lupus erythematosus and rheumatoid arthritis, myocardial infarction, chest trauma, aortic dissection, pancreatitis, irritable bowel syndrome, and some medications, such as procainamide and fibrinolytic agents.

Pathogens that can lead to pericarditis include viruses, such as hepatitis B, varicella and the Epstein-Barr virus. Bacteria like staphylococcus, streptococcus, salmonella and legionella can also lead to the condition, as well as fungi, such as candida, aspergillus, and parasites such as *entamoeba histolytica* and *toxoplasma gondii*.

Signs and Symptoms

Signs and symptoms include a friction rub, a dry cough, low-grade fever, sharp, piercing chest pain over the center and/or left side of the chest, shortness of breath when reclining, weakness, fatigue, and swelling of the abdomen and/or legs. ST-segment elevation in all leads except aVR and V1 is also an indication.

Pericardial rubs are produced by the movement of the inflamed pericardial layers against each other and it is best auscultated upon expiration, when the patient is sitting forward and upright.

Treatment

Treatment for pericarditis varies according to its severity. Mild cases can usually resolve without treatment. Other treatments include pain relief, using a narcotic analgesic or a non-steroidal anti-inflammatory medication (NSAID), corticosteroids, aggressive treatment of the underlying disorder and close monitoring of the patient in terms of cardiovascular status and the presence of complications.

Hospitalization may be necessary if cardiac tamponade occurs. In such cases, a pericardiocentesis may be performed; if the patient is diagnosed with constrictive pericarditis, a pericardiectomy may be necessary.

Peripheral Vascular Disease

Peripheral vascular disease, also referred to as peripheral arterial disease, is a disease that occurs as the result of plaque buildup in the arteries that carry blood to the body. This plaque build-up is known as atherosclerosis. Over time it can accumulate, hardening and narrowing the arteries and limiting the flow of oxygen-rich blood to the organs and other parts of the body.

Signs and Symptoms

Signs and symptoms are not always present, but some experience intermittent claudication, weak or absent pulses, sores or wounds, pale or bluish skin color and erectile dysfunction.

Treatment

Treatments include lifestyle changes, such as quitting smoking, lowering blood pressure, lowering high cholesterol, lowering blood glucose levels, and staying physically active. Other treatment options include medications to treat high cholesterol, lower blood pressure, and prevent blood clots from forming.

Surgery procedures include bypass grafting, angioplasty and stenting, and atherectomy.

Thromboembolic Disease – Deep Vein Thrombosis

Deep vein thrombosis is a blood clot that forms in a vein deep in one's body. Most of the time the blood clots form in the lower leg or thigh; however, they can occur in other parts of the body.

Signs and Symptoms

Only about 50% of the people who have deep vein thrombosis (DVT) experience symptoms, but those who do are typically affected with swelling of the leg, pain, tenderness in the leg while walking or standing, increased warmth in the affected area, and red or discolored skin over the affected area.

Treatment

Treatment includes medications, such as anticoagulants, thrombin inhibitors, and thrombolytic drugs. Other types of treatment include a vena cava filter, when indicated, and graduated compression stockings to increase peripheral venous return.

Gastrointestinal Emergencies

Peritonitis

Peritonitis is an inflammation and infection of the peritoneum that can be caused by a variety of disorders. Peritonitis is most often caused by enteric microorganisms like E. coli following a ruptured appendix or ulcer perforation; however, it can also be caused by gastric secretions entering the peritoneum.

The presence of peritonitis includes white blood cell count is typically elevated to more than 20,000/uL. A paracentesis is sometimes performed to determine the offending microbe and its sensitivity. Ultrasound and abdominal x-rays are also helpful for diagnosis.

Signs and Symptoms

The white blood cell count is typically elevated to more than 20,000/uL. A paracentesis is sometimes done to determine the offending microbe and its sensitivity. Ultrasound and abdominal x-rays are also helpful to the diagnosis.

Some of the signs and symptoms of peritonitis include severe and sudden abdominal pain accompanied by guarding and rebound tenderness, decreased or absent bowel sounds, nausea and vomiting, abdominal distention, fever, malaise, tachypnea and tachycardia, and possible oliguria and shock.

Treatment

Peritonitis is treated with antibiotics and analgesia for pain. Intestinal decompression is used to decrease abdominal distention and to prevent associated respiratory problems. Surgery may be indicated to eliminate the cause, as is the case with a ruptured appendix and other underlying gastrointestinal disorders. The complications of peritonitis include massive sepsis, shock and death.

Appendicitis

Appendicitis is an acute inflammation of the vermiform appendix, which is attached to the cecum. It is a commonly occurring gastrointestinal medical and surgical emergency. It appears to be more common among males, those who consume a low fiber and high carbohydrate diet, and in the younger population, although it can occur among all age groups. Increased morbidity and mortality occurs as a function of advancing age.

Currently, it is believed that appendicitis results from a number of factors including breakdown and damage to the protective mucosal lining of the appendix, which leads to a secondary bacterial infection, rather than a hard mass of feces (fecalith), as was previously thought to be the case. Other possible causes include a tumor, adjacent lymph node edema, parasites and the presence of a foreign body.

This inflammatory process exerts obstructive pressure on surrounding vessels, which engorges the appendix and facilitates the entry for microorganisms and the formation of micro-abscess. If this infection is slow, the body can sometimes temporarily wall off the engorged appendix with a local abscess. In most other cases, appendicitis is a medical emergency that must be treated within 24-36 hours to prevent complications, such as gangrene, perforation or rupture, peritonitis, sepsis, and death.

Signs and Symptoms

The signs and symptoms of appendicitis include the following:

- Characteristic and classic pain in the right lower quadrant of the abdomen (McBurney's point) that may be initially intermittent but becomes steady and severe within a short period

- Tense and rigid abdominal muscles. The person may pull up their knees to relieve pressure on the abdomen

- Rebound tendency and tenderness at Mc Burney's point

- A fever of 100.5° to 101°F will be present, with an elevated white cell count of >10,000/mm3 and neutrophils of >75%.

- Anorexia

- Nausea

- Projectile vomiting

Elderly patients may not demonstrate the classic signs of appendicitis, so clinical evaluation is crucial to making the correct diagnosis.

Abdominal ultrasound, CT scans and white blood cell counts are used for the diagnosis of appendicitis. The white blood cells are elevated (10,000 to 20,000/mm3) and immature white blood cells are indicative of appendicitis.

Treatment

The complications of untreated appendicitis are gangrene, perforation or rupture, peritonitis, sepsis, and death. Postoperative complications can include infection, so treatment is crucial.

The treatment of appendicitis is an emergency surgical appendectomy, which is the complete removal of the appendix. Pain management is implemented during the postoperative course of treatment.

Gastrointestinal Bleeding

Gastrointestinal (GI) bleeding is a definitive sign that there is a problem in the digestive tract. GI bleeding can occur in any of the gastrointestinal organs, which includes the esophagus, stomach, small intestine, large intestine or colon, rectum and anus.

A variety of different conditions cause bleeding in the GI tract. Some are in the upper tract and others are in the lower.

In the upper GI tract, a common cause of bleeding is peptic ulcers, which are open sores that appear in the esophagus, stomach and small intestine. The cause of these ulcers is usually a bacterial infection. Another condition in the upper GI track that causes bleeding is called esophageal varices, which can cause enlarged veins in the esophagus to tear and bleed. Mallory-Weiss tears, which are tears in the walls of the esophagus, is another condition of the upper GI tract that causes upper gastrointestinal tract bleeding.

In the lower GI tract, the most common cause of bleeding is colitis, which is a condition that occurs due to the colon becoming inflamed. Reduced blood flow in the colon, Crohn's disease, parasites, food poisoning or infections could be the cause of this. Other lower GI tract bleeding can occur as the result of hemorrhoids.

Signs and Symptoms

The signs and symptoms of GI bleeding can vary. One of these is dark stools, which can have an appearance similar to tar, and can indicate that the bleeding has occurred in the stomach or upper GI tract. Other signs and symptoms of a gastrointestinal bleed include bright red or burgundy-colored stools, seen when passing a bowel movement, vomiting blood, coffee ground-like stools, hypotension, paleness, weakness, shortness of breath and, when severe, the signs of hypovolemic shock.

Treatment

The treatment for gastrointestinal bleeds includes the following:

- Gastric lavage, which involves a tube being placed through the mouth into the stomach in order to drain the contents of the stomach using intermittent suction

- Esophagogastroduodenoscopy (EDG), which is a thin tube with a camera on the end that is passed through the mouth through the esophagus, stomach and the small intestine to visualize the gastrointestinal tract

- Blood transfusions

- IV fluids and medications

Cholecystitis and Cholelithiasis

Cholelithiasis is the formation of gallstones in the biliary tree. Cholecystitis can be an acute or chronic inflammation of the biliary tree.

Some of the risk factors associated with cholecystitis and cholelithiasis include advanced age, obesity, liver disease, oral contraceptive use, low-calorie diets, rapid weight loss, ileum diseases and disorders, and hypercholesterolemia. Females are prone to these conditions than males, and Hispanic, Native American and Caucasian patients present with them more often than other racial groups.

Most often, acute cholecystitis is caused by a partial obstruction with gallstones, although it can occur without any gallstones present at all. An acalculous cholecystitis usually happens after trauma, surgery or burns. Chronic cholecystitis can cause the gallbladder to turn into a rigid and thickened, fibrotic organ with poor and spastic function.

Signs and Symptoms

The signs and symptoms of cholecystitis are mild gastric distress, epigastric feelings of fullness, particularly after a fatty or large meal, epigastric pain in the right upper quadrant that can be quite severe, biliary colic, Murphy's sign (severe pain when the abdomen is palpated), nausea and vomiting, fever, mild jaundice, a palpable gallbladder and vomiting.

Some of the signs and symptoms of cholelithiasis include upper right quadrant pain, jaundice and other symptoms of biliary colic. Often, it is asymptomatic.

In order to diagnose cholecystitis a radionuclide scan, an endoscopic retrograde cholangiopancreatography and ultrasonography must be performed.

Treatment

Surgery is the treatment of choice. A laparoscopic cholecystectomy is most common but some patients may also be good candidates for extracorporeal shock wave lithotripsy, which disintegrates stones with sound waves. Some pharmacological interventions include ursodiol or chenodiol to dissolve the gallstones. Treatment is crucial to avoid complications that can lead to sepsis.

Liver Cirrhosis

Liver cirrhosis is a relatively common hepatic disorder. It leads to progressive, irreversible and diffuse destruction of the functional parenchyma cells of the liver, which are then replaced with fibrous scar tissue that impairs normal blood flow to this organ.

The three types of cirrhosis are:

1. Alcoholic cirrhosis resulting from alcohol abuse

2. Biliary cirrhosis caused by a biliary tract obstruction

3. Post-hepatic cirrhosis, which is secondary to hepatitis B and C

Although the most common cause of liver cirrhosis is alcohol, it can also be caused by biliary obstructions, toxins, fatty liver disease, hepatitis B and C, and hemochromatosis.

Signs and Symptoms

Although asymptomatic in the earlier stages, cirrhosis results in severe liver parenchyma damage, hepatic dysfunction, and liver failure. Clinical signs and symptoms include ascites, encephalopathy, jaundice, organomegaly, coagulopathy, hematemesis, rectal bleeding, malena, spider nevi, erythema of the palms, gynacomastia, caput medusa, esophageal varices (related to portal hypertension), renal dysfunction and failure (high serum creatinine), and signs of sepsis and shock.

Complications include massive liver failure, multisystem failure and death.

Treatment

Some of the treatments for cirrhosis of the liver include medications, surgery for biliary cirrhosis and dietary management. Dietary sodium, protein and fluids may be restricted.

Some of the medications used include diuretics for ascites, lactulose or neomycin to lower ammonia levels, medications for the control of bleeding relating to esophageal varices (vitamin K, nadolol and isosorbide), iron and folic acid for anemia, and a vasoactive medication like octreotide to reduce portal hypertension.

Some surgical interventions include sclerotherapy for esophageal varices, paracentesis to remove abdominal fluid secondary to ascites and a trans-jugular intrahepatic portosystemic shunt (TIPS) to relieve portal hypertension and ascites. Liver transplantation is the sole cure for cirrhosis of the liver.

Diverticulitis

When one or more diverticula in the digestive tract become inflamed or infected, it is known as diverticulitis. This is most common in people 40 years of age or older.

Signs and Symptoms

Several signs and symptoms can accompany diverticulitis. The most common of these is sudden, severe pain in the left side of the abdomen. Less commonly, they include abdominal pain that increases in severity over several days, abdominal tenderness, change in bowel habits, constipation, diarrhea, nausea and vomiting, bloating, and bleeding from the rectum.

Treatment

A mild attack requires a liquid or low fiber diet and antibiotic, but if the attack is more severe, hospitalization may be necessary to treat any accompanying complications.

Esophageal Varices

Esophageal varices are abnormally enlarged veins located in the lower part of the esophagus. They are normally seen in those with serious liver diseases. These develop when normal blood flow is obstructed by scar tissue in the liver or a clot; due to the blockage, the blood then seeks another route and flows into smaller blood vessels, which may leak blood or even rupture, because they are not able to carry large volumes of blood.

Signs and Symptoms

Unless they bleed, esophageal varices usually have no signs or symptoms. If they bleed, the following may be seen:

- Shock
- Black, tarry or bloody stools
- Vomiting blood

If any signs of liver disease are present, the doctor may suspect esophageal varices. These liver disease signs include jaundice, spider nevi, palmar erythema, Dupuytren's contracture, shrunken testicles, swollen spleen, and ascites.

Treatment

The primary treatment for esophageal varices is to prevent bleeding. This can be accomplished by the use of medications to reduce pressure in the portal vein and by using elastic bands to tie off bleeding veins.

Esophagitis

Inflammation that damages the tissues of the esophagus is known as esophagitis.

Signs and Symptoms

The common signs and symptoms of esophagitis are a decrease in appetite, cough, abdominal pain, vomiting, nausea, food impaction, chest pain (usually behind the breastbone accompanying eating), odynophagia, and dysphagia. In young children, who are often unable to describe their symptoms, feeding difficulties and failure to thrive are common.

Some possible complications occur include esophageal stricture, esophageal rings and Barrett's esophagus.

Treatment

Treatment for esophagitis is aimed at lessening symptoms, managing complications and treating the underlying cause of the disorder.

Gastritis

Gastritis is a response of the stomach's gastric mucosa to infection or injury.

Acute gastritis is an erosive process that commonly results in a gastrointestinal bleed. It is caused by factors such as the ingestion of irritants like alcohol, caffeine, aspirin, NSAIDs and bacterially contaminated foods. An accidental ingestion of an acid or corrosive like lye, Lysol, ammonia and other cleaning agents, radiation therapy, some chemotherapy drugs, shock, major trauma, sepsis and burns are also associated with acute gastritis.

Chronic gastritis can result from an autoimmune response and *H. pylori* infection. Some of the other risk factors associated with chronic gastritis include chronic alcohol use, cigarette smoking and the aging process.

Signs and Symptoms

Gastritis can be asymptomatic or it can be marked with the following symptoms:

- *Acute gastritis:* Anorexia, abdominal cramping, gastrointestinal bleeding, heartburn, melena, diarrhea, nausea and vomiting, fever and epigastric pain

- *Chronic gastritis:* Dyspepsia, anorexia, weight loss, burning epigastric pain unrelieved with antacids and epigastric heaviness after a meal

Serious and life threatening complications include gastrointestinal hemorrhage and shock.

Treatment

Medications used for the treatment of gastritis are antacids, proton pump inhibitors and H_2 receptor antagonists.

Gastroenteritis

Gastroenteritis, which is often mistaken for "stomach flu" by patients, is not actually related to the influenza virus. Gastroenteritis can be mild, self-limiting and resolve in a day or two, or it can be quite severe and long lasting.

One of the most common complications of gastroenteritis is dehydration and associated electrolyte imbalances, which can severely and adversely affect infants, young children and the aging population.

Signs and Symptoms

The signs and symptoms depend upon the severity. Signs include diarrhea, chills, headache, nausea, vomiting, and abdominal pain. More severe cases can have dehydration, bloody diarrhea, and a fever of more than 101 Fahrenheit for more than five days.

Treatment

If the gastroenteritis is caused by a virus, it will usually resolve on its own. Symptomatic treatments include fluids, food as tolerated, and rest to help relieve the discomfort. In more severe cases, dehydration is treated with intravenous fluids and electrolyte replacement, as indicated. If bacteria are the causative agent, antibiotics can be prescribed. Medications such as antiemetics can also be given to help relieve vomiting.

Hepatitis

Hepatitis is the inflammation of the liver. Hepatitis can be acute or chronic and it can lead to serious life threatening liver damage. Although there are many types of hepatitis, viral hepatitis is the most common. Some other types of hepatitis are alcoholic, toxic and hepatobiliary hepatitis caused by alcohol, toxins like acetaminophen and benzene, and cholelithiasis, respectively.

Viral hepatitis can be caused by several viruses and, physiologically, these viruses stimulate an immune response, inflammation and destruction of the hepatocyte cells of the liver.

Signs and Symptoms

Viral hepatitis has three phases, the pre-icteric phase, the icteric phase, and the post-icteric phase. The signs and symptoms of each phase are below.

- *The Pre-icteric Phase*: Signs and symptoms are flu-like and nonspecific complaints like fatigue, anorexia, nausea, chills, fever and mild upper right quadrant pain. Laboratory values indicate elevated urine bilirubin levels, and elevated ALT and AST levels with hepatitis A and B.

- *The Icteric Phase*: During this phase, jaundice, dark urine, clay colored stools, and pruritus occur.

- *The Post-icteric Phase*: The patient begins to feel better during the post-icteric phase of hepatitis. Appetite and activity levels return to near normal.

Treatment

Post exposure to hepatitis A and B is prophylactically treated with immunoglobulins. The treatment of hepatitis, when not prevented, includes vitamin supplementation, vitamin K for prolonged prothrombin times, interferon for chronic hepatitis C, and liver transplantation.

Hernia

When an organ pushes through an opening in tissue or muscle that holds it in place, it is called a hernia. Hernias are most commonly seen in the abdomen, but they can be seen in other parts of the body, such as the thigh, at the umbilicus, and in the groin or inguinal area. The most common type of hernia is the inguinal hernia; other types of hernias include hiatal, umbilical, and incisional hernias.

Some risk factors associated with hernias are genetics, being overweight or obese, a chronic cough, chronic constipation, and smoking. Cystic fibrosis, which impairs lung function, presents with coughing, which may indirectly cause a hernia.

Signs and Symptoms

The most common signs of a hernia include feeling a bulge in the skin, pain and aches in the affected areas, weakness, and pressure or feelings of heaviness. Hiatal hernia symptoms include chest pain, acid reflux and difficulty swallowing.

Treatment

Treatment for hernias can be as easy as a change in diet and monitoring. If the hernia continues to grow and/or it causes severe discomfort, surgery may be necessary.

Inflammatory Bowel Disease

Inflammatory bowel disease consists of two similar but distinct disorders, including Crohn's disease and ulcerative colitis. Both of these gastrointestinal disorders can result from a combination of genetic factors, environmental factors and/or immune system deficiencies. Additionally, both of these disorders are marked with periods of remission and periods of exacerbation.

Some of the differences between ulcerative colitis and Crohn's disease are:

- In those affected with Crohn's disease, the mucosa appears cobblestone-riddled due to granuloma; in contrast, in those affected with ulcerative colitis, the mucosa appears edematous. Shallow ulcerations and superficial bleeding may be visible.

- Crohn's disease generally affects the right colon and distal ileum, while ulcerative colitis generally affects the left colon and rectum.

- Crohn's disease manifests in a noncontiguous and segmented manner; ulcerative colitis manifests in a contiguous and diffuse manner.

- Inflammation in Crohn's disease is transmural; inflammation in ulcerative colitis is mostly mucosal.

Crohn's Disease

Crohn's disease is a chronic idiopathic inflammatory disease that affects the small and large intestines. It is also referred to as ileitis, regional enteritis, granulomatous colitis, transmural colitis, and ileocolitis. Crohn's disease most commonly presents in 30- to 50-year old adults, and Jewish patients of Ashkenazi (Eastern European) descent are at a much greater risk (up to 4-5 times) of developing it than other racial groups. Among non-Jewish patients, the disease more often affects Caucasians, though incidence in African-American patients is increasing.

The intestinal mucosa is thickened and edematous; ulcers in the wall of the intestines form in linear, longitudinal fashion, resembling a cobblestone road. Deep fissures may form in the bowel lining forming a fistula or abscesses. The healing of these abnormalities causes constricted areas in the intestine.

The three phases of Crohn's disease are:

1. The inflammatory phase
2. The fistulizing or perforating phase, and
3. The fibrostenotic (strictures forming during the healing) phase.

Signs and Symptoms

The signs and symptoms of Crohn's disease include abdominal pain and diarrhea as well as steatorrhea, abdominal pain, a palpable upper lower quadrant mass, nausea, vomiting, anemia, weight loss and other symptoms that mimic appendicitis.

Crohn's disease is diagnosed based on signs, symptoms and tests such as a colonoscopy, an upper and lower GI series, trans-abdominal ultrasound, a complete blood count (sedimentation rates are increase during an acute episode), serum albumin, vitamin levels and folic acid levels to determine any malnutrition and/or malabsorption.

Complications include abscesses, anemia, fistulas, perianal disease, gastrointestinal strictures, perforation, anemia and the malabsorption of fat and fat-soluble vitamins.

Treatment

Crohn's disease is treated with medications, dietary changes and surgical interventions when a bowel obstruction is present.

Medications include aminosalicylates, such as sulfasalazine, corticosteroids immunosuppressive agents, antibiotics, monoclonal antibodies, such as infliximab, antidiarrheal agents, acid suppressants, antispasmodics and fat-soluble vitamin supplementation.

Some surgical interventions include segmental resection with anastomosis and strictureplasty.

Ulcerative Colitis

Ulcerative colitis is an idiopathic inflammatory disease of the mucosa and submucosa of the colon and rectum, but it primarily occurs in the distal colorectal area. Ulcerative proctitis is the term for the disease when the rectum is affected.

This disorder continually inflames the area in a diffuse manner, leading to shallow ulcerations and edema. Over time, the area is affected with scar tissue, which leads to a loss of absorption and elasticity of the colon.

Because of its unknown etiology, only the symptoms and effects of the disease can be treated. Some theories indicate that genetics, immune disorders or hypersensitivity disorders are to blame.

Signs and Symptoms

The classic signs and symptoms are abdominal pain and diarrhea. Episodes of diarrhea, which can be mixed with pus, blood and mucus, can occur as frequently as every hour during the acute phase of ulcerative colitis.

Other clinical manifestations include distention of the abdomen, weight loss, iron-deficiency, anemia, fever, dehydration, hypokalemia, nausea and vomiting.

A barium enema will show superficial ulcerations and a narrow pipe-like appearance in the affected area. A flexible colonoscopy will reveal ulcerations of the mucosa and erythema with edema.

Stool analysis will reveal blood and pus when an infectious process is present. The CBC will show anemia, ESR will be elevated, and electrolyte levels will show decreased potassium, magnesium and albumin.

Some complications related to ulcerative colitis include cancer, electrolyte imbalances, perforation with hemorrhage, abscesses, strictures, anal fistulas and toxic megacolon.

A toxic megacolon presents with fever, tachycardia, abdominal distention, peritonitis, leukocytosis, and a dilated colon, which can be visualized with an x-ray. It is life threatening.

Treatment

Medical treatment is supportive and addresses the signs and symptoms. During serious acute phases, the patient may need bed rest, a clear liquid diet, IV fluid rehydration and electrolyte replacement. Total parenteral nutrition is indicated for cases of severe diarrhea to restore a positive nitrogen balance.

Drug therapy can include sulfasalazine (Azulfidine) as the primary medication. Patients allergic to sulfa are treated with oral salicylates such as mesalamine or olsalazine. Corticosteroids, immunosuppressive drugs, purine drugs and antidiarrheal drugs are also used when indicated.

Surgery is performed when toxic megacolon develops and there is a need to rest the colon with a temporary loop colostomy. A subtotal colectomy, an ileostomy, or a Kock pouch procedure can also be performed.

Intussusception

Intussusception occurs when food or fluid is blocked from passing because one part of the intestine slides into another, adjacent part. The affected part of the intestine loses its blood supply, because intussusception cuts it off. Children are at highest risk for intussusceptions.

Signs and Symptoms

The most common symptom in children is pain in the abdomen that causes the infant or child to pull their knees up to their chest. Other signs include stool mixed with blood or mucus, lethargy, lump in the abdomen and vomiting. Less common signs and symptoms include fever, diarrhea and constipation. In adults, abdominal pain followed by vomiting and diarrhea are the most common signs.

Complications include peritonitis and shock.

Treatment

The initial treatment for intussusceptions is to give IV fluids and the insertion of a nasogastric tube. The problem can ultimately be treated with a barium or air enema, and if that does not work, surgery may be necessary.

Bowel Obstructions

An obstruction of the intestinal region is a blockage that keeps food or liquid passing through the small or large intestine. Obstructions can be caused by adhesions formed from surgery, diverticulitis, hernias, and tumors.

Treatment

Treatment for obstructions does depend on the cause of the obstruction, but in most cases, it requires hospitalization.

In addition to tumors in the bowel, other risk factors associated with bowel obstructions are surgical adhesions, fecal impaction, gallstones, the presence of foreign bodies, hematomas, strictures and congenital adhesive banding.

These obstructions can be mechanical and non-mechanical. They can also be complete or partial and incomplete.

Mechanical obstructions occur as the result of adhesions, tumors, intussusceptions, gallstones, volvulus, which is intestinal twisting, hernias, fecal impactions and strictures. Non-mechanical obstructions occur as the result of diminished peristalsis, which can occur with Hirschsprung's and Parkinson's disease.

Waste products and bowel contents accumulate above the obstruction regardless of the cause. This leads to bowel edema and increased capillary permeability, both of which lead to fluid and electrolyte imbalances because the plasma seeps into peritoneal spaces.

Signs and Symptoms

Bowel obstructions lead to increased capillary permeability and bowel edema. These changes lead to impaired fluid and electrolyte balances, vomiting, pain, rigidity, hypotension, tachycardia and fever. Severe complications include bowel gangrene, strangulation, third spacing of fluids, impaired renal perfusion and oliguria.

The table below summarizes the signs and symptoms of large and small intestinal bowel obstructions.

Signs and Symptoms	Small Intestine	Large Intestine
Abdominal Distention	Minimal	Greater distention
Vomiting	Copious and frequent	Rare
Bowel Movements	Less constipation	Pronounced constipation
Pain	Intermittent, cramping colicky pain	Low degree of cramping
Onset	Rapid	Gradual

Treatment

Intravenous fluids and electrolytes are used to treat any fluid and electrolyte imbalances; a nasogastric tube for suction is used to decompress the bowel and antibiotics are sometimes used to prevent infection. Surgical interventions, typically done endoscopically, can eliminate adhesions. Additionally, a bowel resection with re-anastomosis and a temporary colostomy may be indicated.

Pancreatitis

Pancreatitis is an inflammation of the pancreas. There are both acute and chronic cases of this disorder. Some cases can be mild and cured with lifestyle changes but in other situations, pancreatitis can become a serious condition with possible life-threatening complications.

Signs and Symptoms

The signs and symptoms for pancreatitis vary greatly between acute and chronic cases. For acute cases, the patient may experience nausea, vomiting, pain in the abdomen, which increases after ingesting food, abdominal tenderness, pain in the upper abdomen, and pain that radiates from the abdomen to the back.

Chronic pancreatitis can present symptoms such as steatorrhea, weight loss (without trying to lose weight), upper abdominal pain and indigestion.

The complications associated with pancreatitis can be quite serious. They include pancreatic cancer, kidney failure, pseudocysts, malnutrition, infection, diabetes, and breathing problems

Treatment

Initial treatment is focused on reducing inflammation in the patient's pancreas. This usually involves pain medication for the patient, because of the severe pain that is caused by this disorder and abstaining from eating so that the pancreas has an opportunity to recover. Once the inflammation is under control, clear fluids are introduced, and then other foods, as tolerated. Intravenous fluids can help keep the body hydrated.

Once the patient has been initially treated and the pancreatitis is under control, treatment of the underlying disease, or the cause of the pancreatitis, can begin. The treatment varies depending on the type of disease the patient has, but some examples are as follows:

- Gallbladder surgery, which occurs if the cause of the pancreatitis is gallstones; gallbladder surgery includes cholecystectomy (removal of the gallbladder)

- Pancreas surgery, which is performed either to drain the fluid from the patient pancreas or to remove any diseased tissue that may be present.

- Alcohol dependence treatment, which is necessary in some situations, as excessive drinking can cause pancreatitis

- Removal of a bile duct obstruction, as a narrowed or blocked bile duct can cause pancreatitis

Patients who suffer from chronic pancreatitis may require additional treatments such as pain management and pancreatic enzymes, which can be taken in tablet form in order to help the body to digest and process nutrients. A diet that is high in nutrients and low fat can also help ameliorate symptoms.

Peptic Ulcers

Peptic ulcers are the breakdown of the mucous membrane lining of the gastrointestinal tract when it is exposed to gastric digestive juices, pepsin and hydrochloric acid. The mucosal barrier no longer effectively protects the mucosa. Most peptic ulcers are found in the duodenum near the pylorus, although they can also occur in the other areas of the GI tract.

Peptic ulcer disease is more common in men than in women. It also disproportionately affects Hispanics and African-Americans over other racial groups, and is more prevalent in young people.

Current evidence no longer supports the prior thinking that stress and alcohol led to peptic ulcer disease.

The causes of peptic ulcer include *H. pylori* bacteria, non-steroidal anti-inflammatory drugs (NSAIDs), aspirin, corticosteroids, cigarette smoking, Zollinger-Ellison syndrome (a tumor of the pancreas, intestines or stomach that secretes gastrin), and possible genetic factors.

Signs and Symptoms

Some of the signs and symptoms of peptic ulcer disease are:

- Heartburn
- Regurgitation and vomiting
- Dysphagia
- Weight loss
- Anemia
- Tarry black stools (bleeding)
- Evidence of perforation, including:
    - Shallow breathing
    - Shock
    - The absence of bowel sounds
    - A rigid abdomen
    - Pain
    - Pallor
    - Hypotension
    - Cool, clammy skin
    - Tachycardia and other signs of shock and hemorrhage
    - Hematemesis

- o Vomiting blood
- o Pain that can radiate to the back and can occur at night, which is relieved with a meal or snack
- o Hematochezia, which is bright red blood that passes through the rectum with, or without, the presence of stool.

Complications of peptic ulcers include hemorrhage, shock, perforation and GI obstruction.

Treatment

The treatment of peptic ulcers is multifaceted. It includes medications, pain management and possible surgery. Medications include antacids, which reduce pepsin and neutralizer hydrochloric acid, proton pump inhibitors and H2 receptor antagonists, both of which reduce the secretion of gastric acid, as well as antibiotics for *H. pylori*, analgesia and mucosal protective agents like bismuth subsalicylate, sucralfate and misoprostol. Surgery may be indicated when the patient has a perforation. Omental patches and bagotomy are the two primary surgical interventions for peptic ulcers.

Other interventions include the cessation of smoking and avoiding meals before bedtime that appear to increase discomfort.

Stress Ulcers: Curling's and Cushing's Ulcers

There are two kinds of stress ulcers: Curling's ulcers are most common after a massive burn injury, and Cushing's ulcers are primarily associated with traumatic closed head injuries. Pathophysiologically, the gastric mucosa integrity is impaired and broken down as stressors decrease the blood flow to the protective gastric mucosa.

Some of the conditions associated with these stress ulcers, other than head injuries and burns, are mechanical ventilation, shock, sepsis, renal and hepatic failure. Spending time in intensive care also increases a patient's risk for stress ulcers.

Signs and Symptoms

The signs and symptoms, diagnosis and complications associated with stress ulcers are similar to those of peptic ulcers.

There are complications associated with stress ulcers, which include bleeding, shock and death when left untreated.

Treatment

Preventive measures are often highly effective. Patients at risk should be administered antacids, sucralfate and acid suppressors. The patient's gastric pH should be closely monitored and maintained above 3.5 or 4.0.

Genitourinary Emergencies

Urinary Tract Infections

An infection anywhere in the urinary system, including the kidneys, ureters, bladder and urethra, is a urinary tract infection (UTI). UTIs generally appear in the lower urinary tract, or the bladder and urethra. Women tend to suffer from UTIs more often than men do, and these infections can be extremely serious if they affect the kidneys.

Signs and Symptoms

While UTIs may be asymptomatic, symptoms include:

- A strong, persistent urge to urinate
- A burning sensation when urinating
- Passing frequent, small amounts of urine
- Urine that appears cloudy
- Urine that appears red or bright pink (gross hematuria), which is a sign of blood in the urine
- Strong-smelling urine

- Pelvic pain in women

- Rectal pain in men

In older adults, UTIs may be mistaken for other conditions or overlooked altogether.

Different parts of the urinary tract may be infected, so more specific symptoms may indicate different types of UTIs.

UTIs

Part Affected	Signs and Symptoms
Kidneys (pyelonephritis)	- Upper back and side (flank) pain - High fever - Shaking and chills - Nausea - Vomiting - Pus or blood present in the urine - Strong urge to urinate - Burning while urinating
Bladder (cystitis)	- Pelvic pressure - Lower abdomen discomfort - Frequent, painful urination - Blood in urine
Urethra (urethritis)	- Burning upon urination

Treatment

Treatment for a common UTI includes medications, such as sulfamethoxazole-trimethoprim (Bactrim, Septra and others), amoxicillin (Amoxil, Augmentin and others), nitrofurantoin (Furadantin and Macrodantin, among others), ampicillin, ciprofloxacin (Cipro), and levofloxacin (Levaquin).

Pain medication to numb the bladder and urethra may also be prescribed to relieve burning during urination. Additionally, fluids and the monitoring of renal function and urinary output are essential.

Pyelonephritis

Pyelonephritis, a kidney infection, is a specific type of urinary tract infection that begins in the urethra or bladder and travels up into the kidneys. Immediate medical attention is required, because is pyelonephritis goes untreated or is not treated effectively, it can permanently damage renal function and result in sepsis.

Signs and Symptoms

Signs and symptoms include upper back and side (flank) pain, high fever, shaking and chills, nausea, vomiting, pus or blood present in the urine, a strong urge to urinate, and burning while urinating.

Treatment

The first line of treatment is the use of antibiotics, and the type of antibiotic depends on the severity of the infection and the bacteria that are found in the urine. For severe infections, it may be necessary to hospitalize the patient so they can receive intravenous antibiotics.

Epididymitis

Epididymitis is the inflammation and infection of the epididymis, which is part of the male reproductive system. The epididymis is a 6-7 inch tube that connects the efferent ducts from the posterior of each testicle to the vas deferens.

Signs and Symptoms

The signs and symptoms of epididymitis vary according to the cause, but they can include:

- Tender, warm, red or swollen scrotum

- Pain in usually one side of the testicles, which can increase during bowel movements

- Painful and urgent need to urinate

- Pain during intercourse or ejaculation

- Fever and chills

- A palpable lump on the testicle and/or inguinal nodes

- Pain in lower abdomen or pelvic region

- Discharge from the penis

- Blood in the semen (hematospermia)

Treatment

Epididymitis caused from a sexually transmitted infection or any other bacterial infection is treated with antibiotics. If an abscess forms, it is drained; in severe cases, an epididymectomy may be necessary to remove part or all of the epididymis, particularly when there is an underlying physical deformity. It is important to note that even after an epididymectomy, scrotal pain may persist.

Orchitis

Orchitis is an inflammation of one or both testicles. It is most commonly associated with mumps, which is a paramyxovirus. Other causes are bacterial, which can include sexually transmitted diseases, such as gonorrhea or chlamydia. The bacterial form of orchitis usually results from epididymitis, which is referred to as epididymo-orchitis, a combination of the two infections.

Signs and Symptoms

Symptoms, which usually occur suddenly, include swelling in one or both testicles, mild to severe pain, discomfort when sitting, tenderness in one or both testicles that can continue for weeks, nausea, fever, and a discharge from the penis.

Treatment

Bacterial orchitis is usually treated with antibiotics, such as ceftriaxone (Rocephin), ciprofloxacin (Cipro), doxycycline (Vibramycin, Doryx), azithromycin (Zithromax), and trimethoprim and sulfamethoxazole combined (Bactrim, Septra). Ice packs can be helpful to treat the symptoms until the antibiotics start to work.

Treatment for viral orchitis includes pain medication and anti-inflammatory drugs, bed rest, elevating the scrotum and applying ice packs to the area.

Sexually Transmitted Diseases

	Syphilis	Gonorrhea	Chlamydia	Cyto-megalovirus	Herpes Type 2	Group B Streptococcus
Causative Agent	Trepo-nema pallidum	Neisseria gonor-rhoea	Chlamydia trachomatis	Cytomegalovirus	Herpes simplex	Streptococcus group B
Infectious Agent	Bacteria	Bacteria	Bacteria	Virus	Virus	Bacteria
Incubation and Transmission	Usually 3 week, with range from 9 days to 3 months	Men- 3-30 days Women- 3-indefinite		Most common congenital infection; transmitted in utero, labor and in human milk	2 to 20 days. Transmitted during births and in some cases, in utero	
Signs and Symptoms	Primary-chancre(s) Secondary-fever, weight loss, jaundice, rash, alopecia Late-gumma, meningitis, paralysis, paresis, confusion, delusions, impaired judgment slurred speech and tabes dorsalis.	Male - urethritis, dysuria, burning, discharge, painful, swollen testicles Female - discharge, dysuria, burning, feeling of fullness or abdominal or pelvic discomfort vaginal bleeding with intercourse	No signs at times. Female -vaginal discharge, burning with urination, irritation, bleeding after sexual intercourse, lower abdominal pain. Male - urethritis	Often asymptomatic Fatigue, fever, sore throat, and swollen lymph nodes	Vague nonspecific signs like vaginal or urethral discomfort and others such as generalized signs of infection, pain, lesion on the vagina or external genitalia of males.	Often a-symptomatic A urinary tract infection, bacteremia or pneumonia may occur in some cases.
Treatment	Penicillin G	Cipro-floxacin	Azithro-mycin or doxycycline	Valganciclovir, ganciclovir, foscarnet and cidofovir	Anti-viral medications: acyclovir, famciclovir, valacyclovir	Penicillin or another antibiotic

Hepatitis B and C

	Hepatitis B	Hepatitis C
Transmission	Parenteral Sexual Perinatal	Parenteral Sexual Perinatal
Incubation period	4-24 wk	2-20 wk
Virus type	DNA hepadenavirus	RNA flavirs
Diagnostic Serological Tests	*Acute phase*: HBsAg, anti-HBc IgM, HbeAg *Lifetime*: Anti-HBs; Anti-HBc	*Acute phase*: Anti-HDV *Lifetime*: Anti-HCV
Secretions that have been found to contain infective agent	Blood/serous fluids, saliva, semen, urine, nasopharyngeal washings, feces, pleural fluid	Blood, semen
Indication of Protective Immunity	Anti-HBs, total anti-HBc	None
Chronicity	90% infants, 6%-10% adults	50%-80%
Mortality	1%-2%	1%-2%
High-Risk Groups	Household and sexual partners of HBV carriers; immigrants from HBV-endemic areas; IV drug users; patients and staff in custodial care institutions; sexually active gay men; patients on hemodialysis; health care workers with frequent contact with blood	Travelers to endemic areas; people receiving frequent blood transfusions; IV drug users; tattoos; organ transplant recipients; 40% report no risk factors
Vaccine Available	Yes	No

Phimosis

Phimosis is the inability to retract the foreskin of the penis. It is most commonly seen in infants and young children; many cases resolve itself by the age of five years old. Occasionally, it is seen in adults as a result of prolonged irritation or balanoposthitis (inflammation of the glans or foreskin.)

The risk of urinary tract infections, penile cancer, HIV, and sexually transmitted diseases increases in adults with phimosis. In children, the risk factors include urinary tract infections, urinary outlet obstruction, unresponsive dermatologic disease and a suspicion of carcinoma.

Signs and Symptoms

The symptoms can vary in severity. Common symptoms include bulging foreskin, difficulty urinating, inability to pull back the foreskin, pain, and swelling of the tip of the penis.

Symptoms that may indicate a serious condition include paraphimosis, which is a medical emergency that requires immediate care. Symptoms of paraphimosis include discoloration or bruising of the penis tip, a high fever (higher than 101 degrees Fahrenheit), an inability to reposition the foreskin to the un-retracted state, an inability to urinate, and tenderness around the scrotum.

Treatment

Circumcision is the preferred treatment, but betamethasone cream 0.05% bid or tid can be applied to the tip of the penis, the foreskin and the area touching the glands. Betamethasone treatment usually takes three months.

Priapism

Priapism is a prolonged erection of the penis that is not the result of sexual stimulation or arousal. There are two types of priapism. Ischemic priapism is the most common type and is caused by a diminished blood flow from the penis. Non-ischemic priapism is caused by a high flow or abnormally large amount of blood flowing into the penis.

Signs and Symptoms

The signs of ischemic priapism are unwanted erections that last for more than four hours, intermittent erections for several hours (stuttering priapism) and a rigid penile shaft with a soft tip that is painful or tender to the touch. The signs of non-ischemic priapism are unwanted erections that last for more than four hours with the penile shaft erect but not rigid.

Treatment

The treatment of ischemic priapism includes draining the blood from the penis and administering medications such as phenylephrine. This medication can be injected directly into the spongy tissue of the penis to constrict the blood vessels that carry blood to the penis. If these treatments do not work, surgery to implant a shunt may be necessary.

For non-ischemic priapism, the treatment is usually symptomatic since it is often self-limiting. Patients may ice the area and put pressure on the perineum to help stop the erection. In some cases, surgery may be necessary to insert material that temporarily blocks the flow of blood to the penis or to repair arteries or tissue that may have been damaged.

Cancer of the Prostate

Cancer of the prostate is relatively common and often goes unnoticed. Some of the associated risk factors include a family history of prostate cancer, diet, and African American ethnicity. It most commonly occurs in adults over 50 years old.

Signs and Symptoms

The signs and symptoms include dysuria, frequency, pain upon ejaculation, the presence of a urinary tract infection and bone pain in the hips, back or thighs, which is an indication that the cancer has advanced. Diagnosis is made on the results of a biopsy; the most commonly used system for grading prostate cancer is the Gleason score, which ranges from one to ten. A score of one is the least severe, and a score of ten is the most severe and advanced.

Treatment

The treatment of prostate cancer can consist of surgery, chemotherapy, radiation therapy, immunotherapy, and vaccine therapy, depending on the patient's condition.

Prostatitis

Prostatitis is an inflammation of the prostate gland, which can result from an infection. It can be chronic or acute. The types of prostatitis are acute bacterial prostatitis, chronic bacterial prostatitis and chronic nonbacterial prostatitis, which is sometimes referred to as chronic pelvic pain syndrome.

Signs and Symptoms

The signs and symptoms of prostatitis include frequent urinary tract infections, urinary urgency and frequency, pelvic pain, burning upon urination and other signs of infection, such as fever and chills.

Treatment

The treatment of prostatitis includes intravenous antibiotics, pain relief and fluids for the acute bacterial form; fluids and low dose long-term antibiotic therapy can help chronic bacterial prostatitis, and pain relief and fluids are indicated for chronic nonbacterial prostatitis.

Renal Calculi

Renal calculi, also referred to as kidney stones, are small, hard deposits made of mineral and acid salts that form in the kidneys. In some cases, the kidney stone can be caused by hyperparathyroidism.

Signs and Symptoms

Kidney stones do not usually lead to pain until they move around in the kidneys or pass into the ureter. Once the kidney stones begin to move, symptoms can include severe pain located in one's side and back below their ribs, intermittent pain that comes and goes, pain when urinating, pain spreading to the lower abdomen and groin, pink, red, or brown urine, urine that is cloudy or foul smelling, a constant urge to urinate, nausea and vomiting.

The characteristics and intensity of the pain vary as the stones move along the urinary tract. A patient can also have the signs of infection, such as fever and chills, if an infection is occurring along with renal calculi, which is often the case.

Treatment

In addition to symptom relief (particularly pain relief) the treatment varies according to the size of the stone(s). Small stones usually pass by drinking plenty of water and sometimes taking an alpha-blocker.

For large stones, more invasive treatment is often indicated to prevent bleeding, kidney damage and ongoing recurrent urinary tract infections. In some cases, extracorporeal shock wave lithotripsy, which uses sound waves to break up the stone(s) so that they are small enough to pass through the urine, is performed. Percutaneous nephrolithotomy, the surgical removal of the stone, is sometimes required.

Testicular Torsion

Testicular torsion occurs when the spermatic cord that supports the testes in the scrotum is twisted. This twisting cuts off the blood supply to the testicles and surrounding tissue. This can occur at any age, but it is most commonly seen in adolescent males and among neonates during the first week of life.

Signs and Symptoms

Signs and symptoms associated with testicular torsion include lightheadedness, nausea or vomiting, scrotal swelling on one side, blood in the semen, a testicle lump, and sudden pain in the testicle.

Treatment

In most cases, surgery is necessary within six hours of the onset of symptoms to save the testicle. Patients with a history of testicular torsion are at risk of getting testicular torsion in the other testicle in the future.

Urinary Retention

Urinary retention occurs when urine accumulates in the bladder and causes bladder distention. It occurs when the patient is not able to completely empty their bladder and 200 to 250 ml, or 10% of the bladder capacity, is retained. Some of the conditions associated with urinary retention include prostate cancer, benign prostatic hypertrophy, a urethral tumor, neurological dysfunction, trauma and muscular dysfunction.

Signs and Symptoms

Patients with acute urinary retention can experience pain or discomfort, an urge to urinate with no urinary output, abdominal bloating, a weak flow of urine, and urinary leakage between voiding.

Treatment

The treatment often aims to correct and treat the underlying cause. For example, a prostatectomy may be indicated for cancer of the prostate, and a surgical repair may be indicated if the structure and function of the prostate has been damaged by trauma.

Some other treatment interventions include maintaining adequate fluid intake and maintaining normal voiding habits. If these actions aren't successful, a cholinergic drug to stimulate bladder contractions and to facilitate more complete bladder emptying can be used. Crede massage can help a patient with a flaccid bladder. This massage includes manually pressing on the bladder to stimulate emptying.

Urinary catheterization for residual urine may be used, as well as an indwelling urinary catheter, however, whenever possible, catheterization should be avoided in order to prevent UTIs. Catheter-associated urinary tract infections (CAUTIs) are a major concern in healthcare. All invasive procedures and treatments, such as inserting catheters, place the patient at risk for infection. These infections can affect any area of the urinary system, including the bladder, ureters, urethra, and kidney.

The prevention of catheter-associated urinary tract infections includes:

- Inserting and using urinary catheters only when necessary
- The removal of the catheter as soon as possible
- The insertion, care and maintenance of the catheter by only those that are competent to do so
- Maintaining strict aseptic technique
- The use of sterile supplies and equipment
- Maintaining unobstructed urinary flow
- Hand washing
- Maintaining a closed urinary drainage system without disconnecting the catheter from the tubing, or the tubing from the drainage bag
- Securing the catheter to the leg to prevent pulling on the catheter
- Avoiding any kinking or twisting of the catheter
- Always keeping the catheter and bag lower than the level of the bladder to prevent any urinary backflow
- Keeping the bag lower than the bladder to prevent urine from back flowing to the bladder
- Emptying the collection bag frequently and not touching the drainage spout with anything

Some alternatives, like a portable ultrasound device to assess urine volume and antimicrobial-impregnated catheters (such as silver-alloy coated catheters) may reduce the risk for CAUTIs by eliminating the need for catheterization and preventing infection, respectively. Additionally, external condom catheters and intermittent catheterization should be considered for male patients.

Bartholin's Cysts

Bartholin's cysts, which are common, are an obstruction of the Bartholin's glands, which causes fluid to back up into the gland. These cysts can become infected and result in an abscess. A cyst or abscess usually only occurs on one side of the vaginal opening.

Signs and Symptoms

If the cyst remains small and does not become infected there may be no accompanying signs or symptoms, but if it grows it can be felt as a lump or mass near the vaginal opening. If an infection occurs, the symptoms may include painful, tender lump near the vaginal opening, discomfort while sitting or walking, painful intercourse, and fever.

Treatment

Treatments include sitz baths, surgical drainage, antibiotics, marsupialization, and in some rare cases, surgery to remove the cyst if it is not effectively treated with other treatment options.

Vaginal Bleeding and Dysfunction

Vaginal bleeding, a commonly occurring patient's chief complaint when the female presents in the emergency department, can occur among postmenopausal women, non-pregnant women during childbearing years, pregnant women and among young females of all ages.

Abnormal uterine bleeding is defined as vaginal bleeding that occurs other than during the normal menstrual cycle and dysfunctional uterine bleeding is defined as irregular and/or heavy vaginal bleeding that occurs without a known cause.

Abnormal vaginal bleeding is often associated with inter-menstrual bleeding, metrorrhagia, menorrhagia, and post-coital (post intercourse) bleeding. Menometrorrhagia or prolonged and excessive uterine bleeding that occurs irregularly and more frequently than normal, is most often caused by adenomyosis and fibroids, although those with endometrial carcinoma, a problematic intrauterine device (IUD), endometrial polyps, a coagulation disorder and pelvic inflammatory disease are also at risk.

Abnormal vaginal bleeding, among postmenopausal females, must be assessed and managed because it may indicate a malignancy, or a less severe disorder such as vaginitis, atrophic endometritis, endometrial hyperplasia, cervical polyps, and exogenous estrogens.

Vaginal bleeding can be classified as primary dysmenorrhagia, abnormal uterine bleeding and dysfunctional uterine bleeding. Primary dysmenorrhagia is most common among young females.

Signs and Symptoms

Primary dysmenorrhagia is marked with cramping, pain and abnormally excessive flow during menstruation. Other forms of abnormal vaginal bleeding are characterized by unanticipated or excessive vaginal bleeding, which may be accompanied by pain and cramping.

Treatment

If the non-pregnant patient is hemodynamically stable, they are typically assessed and then referred to a gynecologist for possible interventions without emergency treatment.

Primary dysmenorrhagia is treated with an oral contraceptive or non-steroidal anti-inflammatory drugs (NSAIDs), and/or alternative treatments such as a heating pad, exercise, acupuncture, hypnosis, message and/or transcutaneous electrical nerve stimulation using a TENS machine.

Hemorrhage

Some of the most commonly occurring signs and symptoms associated with gynecological emergencies include vaginal bleeding and acute pelvic pain.

Vaginal bleeding, the most commonly occurring patient's chief complaint, can occur in postmenopausal women, non-pregnant women during childbearing years, pregnant women and among young females.

There are several types of vaginal bleeding including primary dysmenorrhagia, abnormal uterine bleeding, and dysfunctional uterine bleeding.

Signs and Symptoms

Primary dysmenorrhagia, most commonly occurring among young females, is marked with cramping and pain during menstruation. Abnormal uterine bleeding is defined as vaginal bleeding that occurs other than during the normal menstrual cycle. Dysfunctional uterine bleeding is defined as irregular and/or heavy vaginal bleeding that occurs without a known cause.

In addition to abnormal vaginal bleeding, other signs and symptoms include post-coital bleeding, adenomyosis, which is a symmetrical enlargement of the uterus, the presence of fibroids, and possible pelvic pain.

Treatment

Primary dysmenorrhagia is treated with an oral contraceptive or non-steroidal anti-inflammatory drugs (NSAIDs), and/or alternative treatments such as a heating pad, exercise, acupuncture, hypnosis, message and/or transcutaneous electrical nerve stimulation using a TENS machine.

If the non-pregnant female is hemodynamically stable, they are typically assessed and then referred to a gynecologist for possible interventions without emergency treatment.

Acute Pelvic Pain

Pelvic/lower abdominal pain is another common reason that women go to the emergency department. This can result from a number of disorders including those affecting the musculoskeletal system, the genital tract, the bowel and/or the urinary tract. At times, acute pelvic pain can result from other causes such as depression, sexual violence, anxiety and domestic violence.

Signs and Symptoms

Pain during the midpoint of the menstrual cycle (*mittelschmerz*) is associated with ovulation. This pain is normal; however, other pelvic pain should be investigated. Pelvic pain is sometimes accompanied by vaginal bleeding.

Treatment

The treatment and management of pelvic pain depends on the etiology of the pain and the diagnosis. At times, a referral to a pain management clinic may be helpful.

Toxic Shock Syndrome

Toxic shock syndrome (TSS) is most frequently caused by *staphylococcus aureus* and streptococcal pathogens. Prior to the changes in tampon manufacturing, toxic shock syndrome was primarily due to tampon use. Now, it is associated with a number of other conditions such as burns, surgery, childbirth and trauma.

Signs and Symptoms

The signs and symptoms of toxic shock syndrome include hypotension, a high fever, scaling and desquamation of the hands and palms of the hands, a diffuse erythematous rash, and multiple system dysfunction and shutdown, which can be fatal.

Renal system effects are signaled by elevated urea nitrogen and creatinine. The neurological system can be affected with changes in the level of consciousness. Other signs and symptoms include the signs of infection, nausea, vomiting and diarrhea.

Treatment

Hospitalization, and even critical care, is typically indicated so that the patient can be treated and monitored in order to reduce the risk of complications and fatality. The patient is given antibiotics and fluids as they are monitored for hemodynamic stability. At times, airway management and drugs to treat refractory hypotension are needed.

The antimicrobial drugs of choice are first generation cephalosporin and penicillin. Vancomycin or clindamycin are used when the patient is allergic to penicillin. Surgical intervention may be necessary to address the cause of the infection, such as an abscess.

Endometritis and Salpingitis

Salpingitis is an inflammation or infection of the fallopian tubes; endometritis is an inflammation or infection of the endometrium. When endometritis is not treated in a timely manner, salpingitis and widespread pelvic inflammatory disease can occur.

Some of the life threatening complications include massive sepsis, the formation of abscesses, and disseminated intravascular coagulopathies. Infertility can also occur.

Signs and Symptoms

Signs and symptoms include diminished bowel sounds, fever, foul smelling lochia, abdominal tenderness, diminished bowel sounds, an elevated white cell count, and tachycardia.

Treatment

Antimicrobial drugs are administered as based on the causative pathogen. Typically, clindamycin or gentamycin are used. Replacement fluids and rehydration, pain control and fever control are initiated as part of the treatment plan. Hospitalization is indicated when the patient is medically unstable, not tolerating oral antibiotic therapy and/or there are indications that the patient is affected with complications.

Pelvic Inflammatory Disease (PID)

The most commonly occurring pathogens that lead to pelvic inflammatory disease are gonorrhea and chlamydia. PID sometimes occurs as a complication of an ectopic pregnancy. Some complications are serious and can cause permanent scarring of the fallopian tubes and infertility if left untreated.

Signs and Symptoms

The signs and symptoms of pelvic inflammatory disease are rebound tenderness, abdominal guarding, acute pelvic pain, vaginal discharge, fever, elevated white blood cell count, post-coital bleeding, and inter-menstrual bleeding.

Treatment

Treatment is based on the offending pathogen and the status of the patient in terms of pregnancy. Non-pregnant females are typically returned home with an antibiotic regimen; pregnant women often are hospitalized to prevent secondary maternal and/or fetal complications. Doxycycline, azithromycin, ceftriaxone, and metronidazole are typical medications.

Tubo-Ovarian Abscess

Tubo-ovarian abscesses can arise as the result of untreated pelvic inflammatory disease and acute salpingitis, as well as with a post-miscarriage, postpartum, or post-abortion infection. Untreated tubo-ovarian abscesses can lead to septic shock and death.

Signs and Symptoms

The classic signs and symptoms include fever, tachycardia, signs of peritonitis, pelvic or lower abdominal pain and foul smelling, bloody lochia.

The diagnosis is confirmed when a pelvic ultrasound reveals fluid in the pouch of Douglas, also referred to as the recto-uterine pouch.

Treatment

Treatment includes broad scope intravenous antibiotic therapy, blood replacement as indicated, and the correction of any fluid and/or electrolyte alterations.

Ovarian Cysts

Ovarian cysts usually occur as the result of a hormonal imbalance. Ruptured cysts can lead to life threatening bleeding or peritonitis.

Signs and Symptoms

Some ovarian cysts are asymptomatic. Others may present with unilateral pain, menorrhagia and/or delayed menstruation. Ruptured cysts can lead to life threatening bleeding or peritonitis after an untreated episode of pelvic or abdominal pain.

Treatment

In most cases, antibiotics and non-steroidal anti-inflammatory drugs (NSAIDs) can help control pain. The patient should be monitored closely in terms of their hematocrit and hemoglobin. In some cases, surgery is indicated.

Blood tests need to be performed. Surgery is not common, but in some cases (especially when hypovolemia is present) it is necessary.

Trauma and Sexual Assaults

Trauma in pregnancy can occur as a result of domestic violence, as well as other events such as attempted homicide, sexual assault and automobile accidents. All traumas to a pregnant women leads to more deleterious effects on the fetus than on the pregnant woman. Some of these are fetal death, *abruptio placentae*, which is the most common cause of preterm labor in the pregnant trauma patient, and uterine rupture.

It is often very difficult to diagnosis domestic violence, especially since many women will not disclose the fact that they have been physically abused. It is essential that emergency nurses interview the victim in a private area and in a sensitive and reassuring manner.

Signs and Symptoms

The emergency nurse will determine whether the pregnant woman is experiencing any contractions, vaginal bleeding, increased vaginal discharge, a backache or abdominal pain. Contractions, vaginal bleeding and abdominal pain can indicate placental abruption, in addition to trauma. Increased vaginal discharge could be amniotic fluid; a backache could signal preterm labor.

Treatment

The primary assessment is related to the ABCs (airway, breathing and circulation). Any shock or hemorrhage is treated and pregnant women should have fetal monitoring for at least for hours when they are more than 20 weeks pregnant.

Threatened/Spontaneous Abortion

A spontaneous abortion or miscarriage is the natural, rather than elective, loss of a fetus prior to the 20th week of gestation. A threatened abortion is a sign that a miscarriage may occur.

Signs and Symptoms

Signs and symptoms include vaginal bleeding with or without cramps, a dull, sharp pain in the abdomen or the lower back, and tissue or clots from the vagina.

Treatment

If the products of pregnancy do not leave the body naturally, the woman should be watched for up to two weeks in order to determine if a dilation and curettage (D and C) is indicated. A medication such as misoprostol may be required in order to remove the contents that remain in the womb.

Ectopic Pregnancy

An ectopic pregnancy is the abnormal fertilization and implantation of the fetus in any area other than the uterus. Most ectopic pregnancies are found in the fallopian tubes.

Signs and Symptoms

Signs and symptoms can include vague and nonspecific complaints such as those associated with GI disorders, like diarrhea and vomiting. The patient may also present with fainting, vaginal bleeding, a history of amenorrhea, and severe abdominal pain. Because some women with an ectopic pregnancy do not even know that they are pregnant, a beta-hCG test should be done on all women of childbearing age who could be pregnant when they appear with the above signs and symptoms.

Treatment

Ruptured ectopic pregnancies are a true medical emergency; some emergency interventions include the correction of hypovolemia resulting from blood loss, and the obstetrician may elect to perform surgery. Anti-D immunoglobulin within 72 hours after any suspected and actual exposure is indicated, and methotrexate may be given for the medical management of un-ruptured ectopic pregnancies.

Emergent Delivery

An emergent delivery is an unexpected, precipitous delivery of a baby, preterm or full term, that occurs or threatens to occur prior to the mother and baby's ability to access standard obstetrical procedures and preparations.

Signs and Symptoms

The signs and symptoms of an emergent delivery are the same signs and symptoms that characterize the final stages of labor including strong, frequent uterine contractions, the maternal urge to push and bear down, a bloody show, breaking water, and the visible crowning of the baby's head in the vagina, or a visible vaginal meatus bulge.

Treatment

The goals of treatment are to ensure the health and wellbeing of the mother and the baby without any complications. The nurse ensures the mother's comfort and the relief of anxiety relating to emergency childbirth.

Treatments and interventions vary according to the amount of time that is anticipated before final delivery. The necessary supplies and equipment, such as Kelly clamps, basins, sterile gloves, respiratory equipment including suctioning and oxygen equipment, bulb syringes and a cord tie or clamp should be readily accessible.

The mother should be encouraged to take deep breaths, do relaxation techniques and *not* push until the appropriate time of labor. The nurse should support the baby's head as it leaves the vaginal canal, remove the umbilical cord if it is around the neonate's neck and clamp the cord with Kelly clamps about two inches apart. The neonate's shoulders should be delivered one at a time, after which the rest of the body is delivered rather easily. After delivery, the neonate should be suctioned to remove any fluid or mucus.

The neonate's Apgar score and vital signs are taken, and the nurse should provide warmth to the mother and baby. The placenta and membranes are retained; the uterus is massaged and frequently palpated in order to keep it contracted during the post-delivery phase and the neonate is placed on the mother's breast if she desires.

Antepartum Bleeding

Antepartum bleeding or hemorrhage is bleeding that occurs from the genital tract during pregnancy.

Signs and Symptoms

- *Sub-chorionic Hematoma* - A sub-chorionic hematoma is a rare complication of pregnancy that occurs when there is a blood clot between the wall of the uterus and the membranes of pregnancy. Bleeding occurs when small areas of the membrane separate from the uterus. There is no known cause for a sub-chorionic hematoma.

- *Hydatidiform Mole* - A hydatidiform mole, also known as a molar pregnancy, is the proliferation of trophoblasts, which leads to the formation of fluid-filled placental areas that appear as a grape-like cluster. Molar pregnancies occur when there is an extra set of paternal chromosomes in the fertilized egg. Because of this abnormality, the placenta grows into a mass of cysts.

- *Incompetent Cervix* - An incompetent cervix, or cervical insufficiency, is a cervix that tends to open too early during pregnancy, thus leading to premature birth. The cervix is closed and rigid in the non-pregnant state. An incompetent cervix begins to soften and open around the fourth or fifth month, which exposes the membrane to the risk of rupture or miscarriage.

- *Spontaneous Abortion* - Types include threatened, imminent, incomplete, complete, missed and septic abortion.

- *Disseminated Intravascular Coagulation (DIC)* - Disseminated intravascular coagulation (DIC) is an acquired clotting factor abnormality. This disorder occurs because of several other underlying conditions, such as an incomplete abortion, retained placenta, a retained dead fetus, an amniotic fluid embolism, and eclampsia. It does not occur as a primary condition; it is always secondary to some other condition or disease. This disorder is somewhat paradoxical, affecting both clotting and bleeding.

Treatment

The treatment of antepartum bleeding includes fluid and blood replacement, as indicated, and other treatments including those that correct the underlying cause.

Hyperemesis Gravidarum

Hyperemesis gravidarum is extreme and persistent nausea and vomiting during pregnancy. A large majority of women experience nausea and vomiting during the first three months of pregnancy, but in some cases, it is so severe that it can result in dehydration.

Signs and Symptoms

Signs and symptoms of hyperemesis gravidarum include severe nausea and vomiting, weight loss, fluid and electrolyte imbalances, lightheadedness, and fainting.

Treatment

Eating small, frequent meals and eating more dry foods can be helpful in the treatment of hyperemesis gravidarum. Drinking plenty of fluids and taking vitamin B6 can also be helpful. In severe cases, it may be necessary to hospitalize the pregnant woman for intravenous fluids and electrolytes.

Neonatal Resuscitation

Neonatal resuscitation is required to some degree in about 10% of neonates at the time of delivery.

Signs and Symptoms

The signs and symptoms include the cessation of cardiac and/or respiratory functioning.

Treatment

The American Heart Association uses the acronym of CAB, which stands for Circulation-Airway-Breathing, for the order of the steps of CPR.

1. Circulation: Restore blood circulation with chest compressions

2. Airway: Clear the airway

3. Breathing: Breathe for the person

Stroke the baby and watch for a response, such as movement, but never shake the baby. If you're the only rescuer and CPR is needed, perform it for two minutes — about five cycles — before calling for help or your local emergency number.

If another person is available, have that person call for help immediately while you attend to the baby.

- *Circulation*: Restore blood circulation. Place the baby on his or her back on a firm, flat surface, such as a table. The floor or ground also will do. Imagine a horizontal line drawn between the baby's nipples. Place two fingers of one hand just below this line, in the center of the chest. Gently compress the chest about 1.5 inches. Count aloud as you pump in a steady rhythm. You should pump at a rate of 100 compressions a minute.

- *Airway*: Clear the airway. After 30 compressions, gently tip the head back by lifting the chin with one hand and pushing down on the forehead with the other hand. In no more than ten seconds, put your ear near the baby's mouth and check for breathing: Look for chest motion, listen for breath sounds, and feel for breath on your cheek and ear.

- *Breathing*: Breathe for the infant. Cover the baby's mouth and nose with your mouth. Prepare to give two rescue breaths. Use the strength of your cheeks to deliver gentle puffs of air, instead of deep breaths from your lungs, to slowly breathe into the baby's mouth one time, taking one second for the breath. Watch to see if the baby's chest rises. If it does, give a second rescue breath. If the chest does not rise, repeat the head-tilt, chin-lift maneuver and then give the second breath. If the baby's chest still doesn't rise, examine the mouth to make sure no foreign material is inside. If the object is seen, sweep it out with your finger. If the airway seems blocked, perform first aid for a choking baby. Give two breaths after every thirty compressions.

Continue CPR until you see signs of life or until emergency personnel arrive.

Preeclampsia and Eclampsia

Eclampsia and preeclampsia are obstetrical emergencies and a leading cause of maternal death.

Signs and Symptoms

Typically, preeclampsia precedes eclampsia; however, this is not always the case. Preeclampsia affects multiple bodily systems and the fetus. It is marked with possible hypertension, proteinuria, and the compromise of one or more maternal bodily systems and/or the baby. At times, there may not be any hypertension. The patient may be normotensive during the initial stages of preeclampsia.

Eclampsia is characterized by seizures that can occur during pre-partum, intra-partum and within 24 hours of the postpartum period. Eclampsia and seizures are often difficult to predict. The woman may be without the following warning signs:

- Proteinuria

- Headache

- Hypertension

- Epigastric pain

- Visual disturbances

The emergency nurse must institute seizure precautions when eclampsia is possible.

Severe hypertension among pregnant women is defined as a systolic blood pressure of 170 mmHg or more and/or a diastolic blood pressure of 110 mmHg or more.

The signs and symptoms of preeclampsia among women after 20 weeks of pregnancy include one, or more, of the following signs and symptoms:

Bodily System or Organ	Signs and Symptoms
Liver	• Severe epigastric or right upper quadrant pain • Increased serum transaminases
Neurological System	• Visual disturbances (photopsia, scotomata, cortical blindness, retinal vasospasm) • Hyperreflexia with sustained clonus • Convulsions when eclampsia is present • Severe headache
Renal System	• Oliguria • Significant proteinuria and a urine protein/creatinine ratio ≥ 30 mg/mol • Creatinine > 90 μmol/L
Hematological System	• Hemolysis • Disseminated intravascular coagulation • Thrombocytopenia
Other Involvement	• Placental abruption • Pulmonary edema • Stroke • Fetal growth abnormalities and arrested growth

Treatment

The treatment of eclampsia includes stopping seizures, treating hypertension with antihypertensive medications and delivery of the baby, if indicated. Magnesium sulfate treats active seizures and it prevents future seizures. Delivery of the baby is the ultimate cure.

HELLP Syndrome

The hallmarks of severe preeclampsia include the triad of symptoms easily remembered as HELLP:

- H- Hemolysis

- EL- Elevated liver enzymes

- LP- Low platelet count

73

Signs and Symptoms

These include elevated liver enzymes, a low platelet count and hemolysis.

Treatment

The treatment of HELLP includes monitoring and the correction of any hematological problems such as low platelets and hemolysis and the treatment of the preeclampsia, as discussed above.

Preterm Labor

Preterm labor occurs when contractions and the cervix begin to open prior to 37 weeks of labor. Preterm labor cannot be stopped.

Signs and Symptoms

The signs and symptoms of preterm labor are sometimes subtle. These include uterine contractions, constant low, dull backache, pelvic and/or lower feelings of pressure, mild abdominal cramps, diarrhea, vaginal spotting or bleeding, water breaking, and a change in vaginal discharge.

Treatment

Treatment options include preparations for the birth of the baby as well as fetal and maternal monitoring.

Fetal Uterine Death

Fetal uterine death can occur as the result of many causes. For example, it can result from a number of preexisting maternal disorders, pregnancy-related disorders and trauma. Some examples of possible traumatic causes include motor vehicle accidents, multiple trauma from explosions, blasts, etc. and domestic violence.

Signs and Symptoms

Fetal death usually presents with the signs and symptoms of a spontaneous abortion, which are abdominal cramping, back pain, and vaginal bleeding.

The diagnosis is made based on signs, symptoms, a speculum examination, ultrasounds, and laboratory tests including human chorionic gonadotropin (hCG).

Treatment

Depending on the severity, intravenous fluids, blood products, dilatation and curettage (D & C) or a suction evacuation may be necessary, particularly when the products of conception are not spontaneously expelled.

Cardiopulmonary Maternal Collapse

Cardiopulmonary maternal collapse is a life threatening medical emergency that can lead to both fetal and maternal death. It can occur as the result of a traumatic injury.

Signs and Symptoms

The signs and symptoms include increases of blood sequestration to the uterus, plasma volume, erythrocyte volume, progesterone mediated tidal volume, cardiac output, oxygen consumption, pulse rate, arterial blood pressure, functional residual capacity, pulmonary wedge pressure, and systemic vascular resistance.

All of the fetuses and maternal bodily systems are compromised with maternal collapse. Death may occur for both the mother and the developing fetus.

Treatment

Immediate treatment with cardiopulmonary resuscitation (CPR) and advanced cardiac life support (ACLS) are essential with complete collapse in addition to early intubation. One modification of CPR for the pregnant woman is that the woman is tilted, or turned, to the left side with a 15° to 30° angle backwards.

Depending on the physical statuses of the mother and fetus and the correction of the underlying cause(s) of the arrest, an emergency caesarean section while the mother is alive or a postmortem caesarean section may be indicated.

Abscess (Peritonsillar)

A peritonsillar abscess is a common bacterial infection of the tonsils that produces a collection of pus. These abscesses usually begin as a complication of untreated, or unsuccessfully treated, strep throat or tonsillitis. It is most common among children, adolescents and young adults, particularly during the winter months.

Signs and Symptoms

Abscesses sometimes appear in the back of the throat as a swollen, whitish blister or boil. Signs and symptoms include infection in one or both tonsils, fever and/or chills, difficulty swallowing or opening the mouth fully, drooling, swelling of face, headache, a muffled voice, sore throat, swollen glands in the throat and jaw, ear pain on the affected side and halitosis.

When severe, the symptoms can also include infected lungs, an obstructed airway, abscess rupture and possible spread of the infection to the mouth, neck and chest.

Treatment

The treatment of peritonsillar abscesses includes antibiotics and a tonsillectomy with recurrent episodes. If not promptly treated, some of the complications can include the spread of infection, pneumonia and bacterial infections affecting the heart and lungs.

Dental Conditions

At times, patients may present in the emergency department with complaints of pain relating to tooth decay (dental caries) and gum disease or gingivitis, which is the inflammation and infection of the gums. These minor cases are typically referred to a local dentist for treatment and the relief of pain.

Other dental conditions that require emergency care include those associated with dental and oral trauma. Dental trauma can result from injuries that occur to the tooth, such as occurs with tooth crown and root fractures, as well as traumatic injuries that affect the periodontal or supporting tissues of the mouth. These injuries include luxation injuries like tooth displacement and tooth avulsion, and tooth subluxation injuries, which loosen a tooth or multiple teeth.

Avulsion Injuries

Dental avulsion is the traumatic loss of a tooth. It can occur as the result of any major or minor trauma such as an assault, auto accident, blast injury or a contact sports injury that affects the mouth.

Signs and Symptoms

The loss of a tooth, bleeding and pain are the signs of a dental avulsion.

Treatment

Dental avulsion is a true dental emergency. The goal of treatment, whenever possible, is to restore and re-implant the tooth. Avulsed teeth in the field should be placed in cold milk as soon as possible and transported to the emergency department. Periodontal ligament cells are not viable when they are left dry and not placed in milk or normal saline. The avulsed tooth should only be handled by the crown portion of the tooth. After re-implantation, splinting helps ensure successful recovery. Avulsed deciduous teeth, also called milk or baby teeth, are not re-implanted because of the risk of damaging underlying, developing permanent teeth.

Luxation Injuries

Luxation injuries are injuries that result when part of the tooth, and not the entire tooth, is moved from its socket.

Signs and Symptoms

Luxation injuries are visible to the naked eye, and accompanied by pain and bleeding.

Treatment

Luxation injuries of permanent teeth are treated with repositioning using firm pressure while the patient is under local anesthesia. Splinting against the adjacent sound teeth using either glass ionomer cement (GIC) powder alone or a combination of GIC and fine wire is indicated. Other splinting options are a mouth guard or orthodontic retainer. Like avulsions, there is no attempt to reposition deciduous teeth; however, the tooth is extracted to prevent aspiration of the loose tooth.

Epistaxis

Epistaxis, or a nosebleed, is a nasal hemorrhage that can be very dramatic and anxiety-provoking. Although cases are usually minor and easily treated, epistaxis can be life threatening, particularly among the elderly and patients on anticoagulants.

Epistaxis occurs more often during the winter months because dry, cold air dries the normally moist nasal mucosa. The pediatric population is at greatest risk because they tend to place foreign bodies into the nasal passage, and pick their nose.

Signs and Symptoms

These include bright red blood and bleeding from the nasal passages. A posterior area nosebleed is when the patient can feel blood running down their throat; an anterior area nosebleed is characterized by the presence of blood in one nostril.

Treatment

After assessing the airway, breathing and circulation of the patient, treatment includes the application of uninterrupted and firm pressure beneath the nasal bone, or Little's area, for approximately fifteen minutes. Multiple attempts may be necessary. The patient should be upright with their head forward in order to avoid the possibility of swallowing blood, which can cause the patient to vomit and dislodge a recently formed clot.

Other treatments can include cauterizing the vessel, nasal packing, and the placement of a large bone cannula or balloon catheter to stop bleeding. Analgesia may be administered to the patient because some of these interventions are painful.

Bell's Palsy

The facial nerve controls facial expressions, tears, taste, and to some extent, hearing. Bell's palsy is a complete or partial weakness of the facial nerve that typically occurs suddenly and without warning in less than 48 hours. Pregnant women, people with diabetes, influenza, a cold, or other respiratory illnesses are at greatest risk for Bell's palsy. It can occur at any age.

Signs and Symptoms

These include a crooked smile, slurred speech, facial numbness or tingling, a "pulling" sensation in the face where the face or mouth feels like it is pulling to one side, teary or dry eye, sensitivity to loud sounds, difficulty eating, headache, pain behind the ear, and a change in the taste of foods.

Treatment

The vast majority of patients with Bell's palsy recover without any treatment; it is primarily self-limited. Other patients may be treated with steroids, such as prednisone or methylprednisolone, to reduce nerve inflammation, which can improve facial nerve recovery. Eye care is important in case of paralysis of the eyelid in order to prevent debris from entering the eye, as normally occurs with blinking. Moistening eye drops are used for dry eyes and the absence of blinking because these symptoms can cause corneal abrasions.

Facial nerve decompression surgery may be done to remove pressure; other surgical options to improve the appearance and function of the face are eyelid surgery, facial nerve grafts, suspension techniques or brow/face lifts.

Foreign Bodies in the Ear

Emergency nurses frequently encounter patients with a foreign body in their ear. It is more common among the pediatric, rather than the adult, population because children are more prone to putting foreign bodies into orifices and openings like the nose and the ear. These can range from a small toy, bead or button to a live insect.

Signs and Symptoms

A child may be completely unaware of the exact nature of the problem. Children may also consciously withhold information for fear of punishment. Itching or discharge can accompany a foreign body lodged in the ear. When an insect is lodged in the ear, the patient may hear a buzzing sound. An auroscope is used to visualize the foreign body and determine whether the tympanic membrane is traumatized, or perforated.

Treatment

The removal of a foreign body from the ear can be risky and challenging to prevent further trauma and injury such as bleeding and inflammation. Physician ENTs are typically called on to perform the removal process.

If the patient has round and smooth item lodged, a hook or gentle suction is used. A patient that presents with organic matter in the ear, such as cotton wool or paper, typically present with additional problems because these organic materials tend to swell, making it more difficult to remove the object or flush it out. Crocodile forceps are often used. After a foreign body has been removed, the ear is reexamined with an auroscope to determine whether any debris remains and to assess for any further ear damage that resulted from the removal of the foreign body.

Discharge education should address the causal factors of the foreign body lodgment. For example, parents and legal guardians should be taught how to "baby proof" their home so future problems can be prevented. Adults, on the other hand, should be instructed to avoid placing objects in the ear (including proper Q-tip use.)

Foreign Body in the Nose

Like foreign body lodgment in the ear, children are at greatest risk for foreign bodies in the nose.

Signs and Symptoms

The object can often be visualized by the parent and/or the emergency department nurse. Unilateral nasal discharge and pain are common signs and symptoms.

Treatment

An older child may be able to remove the foreign body by blowing out of the affected nostril while occluding or pinching off the unaffected nostril. Aspiration may occur during this attempt when the patient inhales rather than blowing out the foreign body. The object may lodge further into the nose and cause more damage.

An alternative method is forceps removal; the nasal passage is sprayed with a local anesthetic spray, after which the object is removed with a forceps. The child may be sedated in order to safely perform the procedure when the child is in distress or is uncooperative. Like the ear after removal, the nose is also thoroughly reexamined after the removal to determine if there is any damage inside the nasal cavity and to determine if all debris and objects have been removed.

Ludwig's Angina

Ludwig's angina is a bacterial infection on the floor of the mouth under the tongue that often develops after a tooth infection, such as an abscess or an oral trauma.

Signs and Symptoms

These include swelling, which may block the airway or impair swallowing, drooling, pain, earache, fever, neck pain and swelling, weakness and fatigue.

Treatment

Treatment may include a breathing tube or tracheostomy if the swelling blocks the airway. Antibiotics, initially given intravenously, can be prescribed to treat the infection. Dental treatment may be necessary if a tooth infection is the cause. Surgery may be required to drain the fluids when swelling is excessive.

Otitis Externa

Acute otitis externa can be caused by trauma, a fungal invasion, and from chemicals and/or excessive moisture in the ear canal. For example, the ear canal can be traumatized with a foreign body like a Q-tip, a buildup of earwax or a small toy; it also results from chemicals and swimming ("swimmer's ear").

Signs and Symptoms

Patients with otitis externa present in the emergency department with complaints of itching, muffled hearing and ear pain that can be very severe, particularly when the jaw is opened or the pinna is moved.

Treatment

The components of care include suctioning using direct visualization. Ear syringing with water is NOT recommended. Pain is treated with an analgesic such as ibuprofen;

a combination of antibiotic/corticosteroid eardrops can be used for bacterial infections. Fungal infection requires a longer course of treatment.

Acute Otitis Media

Children less than ten years old are at greatest risk for acute otitis media because of their age-related ear anatomy, but it can occur at any age. Acute otitis media is an inflammation and infection of the middle ear posterior to the eardrum, or tympanic membrane. It often follows an upper respiratory infection.

Signs and Symptoms

Auroscope examination reveals redness and swelling, bulging of the tympanic membrane and a tympanic membrane that is lumpy and colored red or yellow; this membrane is normally smooth and pink. Other signs and symptoms include coughing, a sore throat, dysphagia, tugging at the earlobes, irritability, pain, crying, fever, headache, tachycardia, malaise, and ear discharge.

Treatment

Many cases of acute otitis media are self-limiting without the use of antibiotics such as amoxicillin. Pain is treated with an analgesic, such as ibuprofen, and the application of heat over the affected ear to reduce swelling and facilitate the reabsorption of excessive fluids.

Mastoiditis

Mastoiditis is a very serious infection of the middle ear's mastoid bone, which can lead to adverse complications including the spread of the infection to the brain. Mastoiditis most commonly occurs following a middle ear infection like otitis media and among children. Some can have a chronic form of mastoiditis, which is marked by ongoing infections and persistent ear drainage.

Signs and Symptoms

Some of the signs and symptoms are pain, tenderness, swelling and redness around the mastoid process, fever, irritability, ear drainage and a displaced pinna that has moved away from the side of the head.

Treatment

Treatment must be swift to prevent serious life threatening, intracranial infections like meningitis, as well as permanent hearing loss. Intravenous antibiotics, a surgical drainage of the abscess (myringotomy), or a mastoidectomy, which is the surgical removal of the infected parts of the mastoid, are sometimes indicated.

Sinusitis

Acute and chronic sinusitis, also referred to as rhinosinusitis, are infections of the sinuses. Chronic sinusitis can be caused by infection, nasal polyps or by a deviated septum, and is usually seen in young to middle-aged adults.

Signs and Symptoms

Signs and symptoms include inflamed and swollen sinuses, a thick, yellow or greenish discharge drainage from the nose or down the throat, headache, aching in upper jaw and teeth, halitosis, fatigue, fever, coughing, an impaired sense of taste and smell, nasal obstruction and congestion, pain, tenderness and swelling around the eyes, cheeks, nose or forehead.

Treatment

Treatments include saline nasal spray, nasal corticosteroids, decongestants, and over-the-counter pain relievers. For severe cases of bacterial sinusitis, antibiotics such as amoxicillin or doxycycline may be indicated.

Labyrinthitis

Labyrinthitis is an inflammatory or non-inflammatory disorder of the labyrinth in the inner ear. The labyrinth transmits information to the brain relating to the movement and position of the head. Faulty information from the labyrinth leads to the person feeling as if they are spinning and dizzy, or as if they are suffering "sea sickness".

Signs and Symptoms

Labyrinthitis typically occurs abruptly, without warning. Patients often think that they are experiencing a stroke or a brain tumor because of the dizziness. The most common symptoms of labyrinthitis are vertigo, nausea, vomiting, a loss of balance, headache, tinnitus or ringing in the ears, rushing noise in the ears and hearing loss that worsens when the patient moves their head, sits up, looks up and/or rolls over.

Treatment

Labyrinthitis is treated symptomatically. For example, the patient may be given antiemetics to control vomiting and/or a motion illness medication like Dramamine to control vertigo. Upon discharge, instruct the patient to avoid driving, heights and operating heavy equipment until one week has passed without any symptoms. The patient should drink plenty of fluids to avoid dehydration secondary to vomiting.

Meniere's Disease

Meniere's disease affects the inner ear, and is seen most often among people in their forties and fifties, although it can occur at any age. Usually, it affects only one ear.

Signs and Symptoms

The signs and symptoms of Meniere's disease include vertigo, often accompanied by nausea and vomiting, hearing loss, tinnitus, and a feeling of fullness or increased pressure in the ear. Episodes often occur in clusters with long periods of remission between the episodes.

Treatment

There is no cure for Meniere's disease, so treatment is aimed at managing symptoms and their severity. Medications such as Antivert or Valium reduce the vertigo, nausea and vomiting. Anti-nausea and antiemetic drugs can be used, and long-term diuretics as well as fluid intake restrictions decrease fluid volume and pressure in the ear. In severe cases of vertigo, a surgical endolymphatic sac procedure, a shunt, vestibular nerve section, or labyrinthectomy may be indicated.

Ruptured Tympanic Membrane

A ruptured tympanic membrane can result from trauma or an infection. Pressure in the middle ear causes the tympanic membrane to rupture. Some examples of trauma are being slapped over the ear, inserting a Q-tip into the ear to clean it, being in the vicinity of an explosion, and non-penetrating traumatic injuries that occur with things like altitude changes, skydiving, and scuba diving.

Signs and Symptoms

A patient presenting with this disorder typically experiences discharge from the ear, sometimes bloody, as well as severe ear pain and hearing loss in the affected ear.

Treatment

The treatment of a ruptured tympanic membrane varies. If the tympanic membrane has ruptured because of a foreign body, this is removed; if the cause is a bacterial infection, antibiotics are is recommended. Pain is managed with an analgesic.

The patient should be advised to keep water out of the affected ear canal and to use analgesics to manage the pain. These ruptures will usually heal in a matter of a few months. Follow up care with an ear/nose/throat (ENT) physician is recommended.

Temporomandibular Joint (TMJ) Dislocation

The temporomandibular joint (TMJ) is a paired synovial joint that is capable of both hinge and sliding movements.

Signs and Symptoms

Patients with TMJ dislocation present with an opened mouth, anxiety and pain.

Treatment

Manual pushing of the mandible downwards and backwards can reduce the dislocation. Both hands are placed on the lateral border of the mandible, with the thumbs on the outside surface of the teeth, after which the mandible is pushed downwards and backwards so the condyles move back into the fossa.

A muscle relaxant, such as diazepam, may be necessary if the muscles spasm. A general anesthetic may be necessary for more severe cases, and anti-inflammatory medication is indicated for pain relief.

Ear and Ear Lobe Trauma

Trauma to the earlobe and ear can occur during a sporting event, an assault or with an accidental introduction of a sharp object. At times, a sub-perichondrial hematoma between the perichondrium and the cartilage may be present.

Signs and Symptoms

An auroscope should be used to inspect the ear and ear canal for possible injuries. Depending on the location(s) of the injury and its severity, the patient may exhibit pain, bleeding, hematoma, lacerations, internal ear damage and signs of trauma.

Treatment

Ear lobe trauma is treated according to its nature and severity. Direct pressure should be used to stop any bleeding that may be present. While inspecting drainage from the ear, the emergency nurse must be able to differentiate among sanguineous or bloody discharge, serosanguineous discharge and cerebrospinal fluid, which is a clear liquid and indicative of severe brain injury. A patient with a superficial laceration is treated by applying a non-pressure dressing and cleaning the affected area(s) with normal saline. At times, reconstructive or cosmetic surgery is done to restore the normal appearance of the external ear structures. All patients are encouraged to follow up with their physician within 24 hours of discharge to the home to ensure proper healing and the prevention of infection.

When a patient has a sub-perichondrial hematoma, this blood causes pressure on the cartilage, which can lead to tissue necrosis. It is treated with the evacuation of the blood followed by a pressure bandage in order to prevent any re-accumulation. This disorder can result in "cauliflower ear" if left untreated.

Nose Trauma

Nose trauma can result from any accident, assault or contact sports.

Signs and Symptoms

The internal aspect of the nose is thoroughly examined with a nasal speculum. Signs and symptoms include pain, epistaxis, facial ecchymosis, and nasal discharge. The leakage of cerebrospinal fluid from the nostrils indicates an orbital blow-out fracture.

Treatment

Patients with facial trauma are assessed by the emergency nurse. This assessment consists of a physical examination and the history of the nose trauma. After the ABC's and any life threatening injuries are assessed for and treated, the nose is treated.

When a patient suffers a trauma to the face, their head should be kept elevated and first aid measures such as applying ice to the site of the injury are done in order to decrease any swelling. When there is the suspicion of a possible nasal fracture, speculum examination may reveal an abnormal appearance of a cherry-like structure, which is an indication of septal hematoma. Deforming infection and necrosis of the nasal cartilage can occur if nasal trauma is left untreated. An ENT specialist will usually perform an incision and drainage to treat any infections.

Patients must be informed about their need to follow-up with an ENT seven to ten days after the initial injury and discharge from the emergency department.

Ocular Emergencies

Ocular Airbag Injuries

The introduction of airbags in automobiles in the 1970's, although instrumental for decreasing injuries and fatalities, has increased the incidence of injuries to the eye(s).

Signs and Symptoms

Several types of injuries can result from a deployed airbag. They include contusions, abrasions, lacerations, retinal tears and detachments, hemorrhage, thermal burns, blindness, bulbus oculi which is the separation of the eyeball from its appendages, orbit, and alkaline burns to the eyes from the airbag's nitrogen.

Treatment

An ophthalmologist examines the patient's eyes and treats injuries, as indicated.

Corneal Abrasion

Some of the many causes of corneal abrasion are deployment of an airbag, a foreign body in the eye, fingernail scratching, abnormal eyelid positioning (entropion, ectropion), explosions, traumatic facial nerve damage that leads to poor or absent blinking, contact lens use, and abnormal eyelashes (trichiasis).

Signs and Symptoms

Patients with corneal abrasions report a feeling that that they have something in their eye. Tearing, a red eye, blurred vision, headache and sensitivity to light are some of the signs of a corneal abrasion.

Treatment

Most corneal abrasions will heal within 24 to 48 hours. Contact lens wear can be continued after two or three days in most cases. Patients with recurrent corneal abrasions should seek treatment from an ophthalmologist to determine if there are any treatable underlying problems.

Ocular Burns

Chemical burns can occur from acids, alkali chemicals, alcohol and solvents. Burns involving more than one-third of the epithelium and the corneal edge are the most serious, particularly when there is corneal clouding.

Signs and Symptoms

Signs and symptoms include clouding of the cornea and corneal melting.

Treatment

Immediate treatment includes irrigation with an intravenous set and a continuous flow of normal saline or Ringer's lactate. This irrigation should be continuous and last for at least 30 minutes or even longer with some injuries like limbus ischemia.

Alkaline burn treatment is done with 10% citric and ascorbic drops q 2h for at least 48 hours and up to one week in combination with 1 g ascorbic acid orally each day. This treatment prevents melting of the cornea. Topical antibiotics like chloramphenicol and steroids, like prednisolone, are used to decrease the inflammatory process and further damage.

Corneal Foreign Bodies

Corneal foreign body injuries can result from accidents, usually on-the-job.

Signs and Symptoms

Patients experience eye irritation, pain and redness. Unless the foreign body is lodged at the center portion of the cornea, there is no effect on visual acuity.

Treatment

In order to remove a corneal foreign body, a topical anesthetic is applied and the foreign body can be removed with moistened Q-tip while using a slit lamp. An ophthalmologist should be consulted for the removal of any foreign body that is central and/or deep, as it has the risk of causing perforation and/or corneal scarring. When a metallic foreign body is in the eye, corneal rusting is a possible complication. When treating a patient with this type of injury, use a combination of antibiotic ointment and padding for twenty-four hours in order to loosen the foreign body so it can be removed easily with a fine hypodermic needle. Eye drops such as cyclo-pentolate 1% or homatropine 2%, which are short acting drops, help relieve pain.

Glaucoma

Glaucoma is a group of diseases that results in damage to the optic nerve. The cause in most cases is abnormally high intraocular pressure. The two most common types of glaucoma are primary open-angle glaucoma and angle-closure glaucoma.

Signs and Symptoms

The signs and symptoms of the two common types of glaucoma are different. With primary open-angle glaucoma there is a loss of peripheral vision that occurs gradually (usually in both eyes) and as the disease advances, tunnel vision occurs. Acute angle-closure glaucoma signs and symptoms are pain, nausea and vomiting, blurry vision, halos around the eye and redness. Acute angle-closure glaucoma is an emergency.

Treatment

Emergency treatment for acute angle-closure glaucoma is aimed at lowering intraocular pressure. This usually requires both medication and a laser peripheral iridotomy, a procedure in which a small hole is made in the iris to allow aqueous humor to exit through the hole, thus decreasing intraocular pressure.

Conjunctivitis

Conjunctivitis, also referred to as pink eye, is an inflammation or infection of the eyes' conjunctiva. When the small blood vessels in the conjunctiva become inflamed, they are more visible, which is what causes the whites of the eye to appear reddish or pink. It is most commonly caused by a bacterial or viral infection. In babies, the cause can be an incompletely opened tear duct.

Signs and Symptoms

The most common signs and symptoms that occur with conjunctivitis, which can occur in one or both eyes, include redness, itchiness, tearing, a feeling of grit in the eye and discharge that can crust during sleep, making it difficult to open the eye(s).

Treatment

Treatment for bacterial conjunctivitis is an antibiotic eye drop or ointment. For viral conjunctivitis, there is no cure, but if caused by herpes simplex, antiviral medications may help. Treatment for allergic conjunctivitis includes eye drops and medications like antihistamines, mast cell stabilizers, drugs to treat inflammation, and steroids.

Iritis

Iritis is an inflammation that affects the iris of the eye; it is a type of uveitis, sometimes referred to as anterior uveitis. A serious condition if left untreated, it can lead to glaucoma and the loss of vision. Iritis can be chronic or acute.

Signs and Symptoms

The signs and symptoms of iritis include eye redness, discomfort or achiness in the affected eye, photophobia, blurred vision, and floaters or spots in the vision.

Treatment

The treatment of iritis is aimed at pain relief and vision preservation. Treatment most often includes steroid eye drops and/or dilating eye drops, but if symptoms don't clear up, oral steroids or other anti-inflammatory drugs are indicated.

Retinal Artery Occlusion

A blockage in one of the arteries that carry blood to the retina is known as retinal artery occlusion. The cause of the blockage can be a blood clot that travels to the eye from other parts of the body such as the carotid artery. These blockages are common among patients with ocular atherosclerosis, temporal arteritis, IV drug abuse, hypertension, hyperlipidemia, atrial fibrillation, diabetes and carotid artery disease.

Signs and Symptoms

Signs and symptoms include a sudden, complete blurring of vision in one eye, which is known as central retinal artery occlusion, or in part of one eye, which is known as branch retinal artery occlusion. A retinal artery occlusion can last for a few seconds, minutes or it can be permanent.

Treatment

No treatment for visual loss affects the whole eye unless caused by a treatable underlying disorder. Retinal artery occlusions can signal the presence of clots in other areas of the body, which can be life-threatening when undiagnosed and untreated.

Retinal Detachment

A retinal detachment occurs when the retina of the eye peels away from its underlying layer of support tissue. Normal function of the retina is to perceive light and to send an impulse to the optic nerve. Retinal detachment may be spontaneous or it can follow trauma. The condition is usually unilateral, and it is a medical emergency. Without immediate treatment, the initial detachment, normally localized and small, can completely detach and lead to complete visual loss and blindness.

When the retina is torn, loss of blood and oxygen supply renders the retina unable to perceive light. Sometimes a small tear, known as posterior vitreous detachment, can be caused by an injury or trauma to the eye or head. With this traumatic injury, the vitreous membrane separates from the retina, thus allowing the vitreous fluid to seep through under the retina and peel it away.

Signs and Symptoms

There are various different signs and symptoms associated with a retinal detachment. Patients will often complain of flashing lights, floaters and a veil or curtain coming over their visual field. Retinal detachments are commonly preceded by a posterior vitreous detachment, which is characterized by symptoms such as photopsia (perceived flashes of light), heaviness in the eye and a sudden increase in the amount of floaters, particularly in the temporal area of the visual field.

Treatment

Treating detached retinas focuses on finding and closing the breaks that have formed in the retina. The principles of treatment include finding all retinal breaks and the prevention of vitreoretinal traction. Most cases are successfully treated with one surgical intervention if surgery is necessary, but others may require more operations.

Over a period of a few weeks, many patients will gradually regain their vision; however, their visual acuity may not be as good as it was prior to the detachment, especially in those cases where the macula was involved.

Hyphema

Hyphema is bleeding in the anterior (front) chamber of the eye, located between the cornea (the front clear surface of the eye) and the iris (the colored part of the eye.) Hyphema is caused by external compression and secondary expansion of the angle in the anterior portion of the eye where the cornea and iris join.

The most common causes of hyphema are blunt trauma and intraocular surgery. Initially, blunt trauma to the eye can cause a small hyphema, but it can advance to severe bleeding over the next three to five days. These types of blunt trauma injuries are caused, for example, by an injury sustained during a sport, falls and fights.

Spontaneous hyphema can also occur; this is usually caused by the abnormal growth of blood vessels (neovascularization) or eye tumors like retinoblastoma, rubeosis iridis, myotonic dystrophy, leukemia, hemophilia, uveitis, juvenile xanthogranuloma and von Willebrand disease.

Signs and Symptoms

Hyphema can appear as a small pool of blood in the cornea or at the bottom of the iris that appears with a reddish colored tinge to the eye. A small hyphema may not be visible to the naked eye, but a larger hyphema may look as though the eye of the patient is filled with blood. A patient suffering from hyphema can experience symptoms such as pain, blurry vision, the loss of vision and/or sensitivity to light.

Treatment

All hyphemas need to be assessed and treated by an ophthalmologist.

The grading system for hyphema is as follows:

1. The blood level is less than 1/3
2. The blood level is greater than 1/3 but less than 2/3
3. The blood level is greater than 2/3 but less than total involvement
4. The blood level fills up the entire anterior chamber

All hyphema is assessed and treated by an ophthalmologist to prevent permanent visual impairment. The intraocular pressure that increases due to blood accumulation can remain high for almost a week before it drops back down to its normal level.

The main goal of treatment is to decrease the risk of continued bleeding, corneal bloodstaining and atrophy of the optic nerve. The patient is instructed to elevate their head at night, to wear a patch and shield covering the affected area. Cases that do not resolve with pressure-controlling medications may require surgery to rid the blood in the anterior chamber of the eye and to prevent corneal bloodstaining. For pain management, acetaminophen can be used; aspirin and ibuprofen should not be used because of their anticoagulant effects.

Eyelid Lacerations

Eyelid lacerations can be caused by numerous types of blunt and penetrating facial traumas. Eyelid lacerations can be extra-marginal and cause tissue loss; they can also involve the lid margin, which requires meticulous suture techniques to repair.

Signs and Symptoms

It is important to check for other ocular injuries that may be present because superficial signs may mask deeper lacerations. This is especially true in children, because they are usually unable to give complete health histories. Assume that any full thickness eyelid laceration is a penetrating ocular injury or a ruptured globe until proven otherwise. A CT scan and X-ray can help to assess for any foreign bodies or fractures that may be present, whether they may be corneal, orbital or intraocular.

The signs and symptoms that accompany conjunctive lacerations are pain, redness, and the feeling that something foreign is in the eye. Lacerations to the cornea and the sclera have accompanying symptoms such as pain and decreased vision.

Treatment

Some treatments for eyelid lacerations include irrigation, debridement to remove foreign material and dead tissue to prevent infection and promote healing. The laceration should be sutured with #6/0 non-absorbable sutures, with removal in three to five days. The patient should keep their head upright at a thirty-degree angle and use cold packs on the affected area to decrease swelling. Applying chloramphenicol ointment will help treat the laceration, and follow up care with an ophthalmologist is required so any lid notching can be assessed and treated.

Nasolacrimal Tearing and Laceration

Nasolacrimal lacerations, also referred to as epiphora, are tearing of the lacrimal or tear ducts that typically occur with traumatic injures, including nasoethmoidal, nasal and mid-facial fractures.

Signs and Symptoms

These include accumulation of mucopurulent discharge and possible conjunctivitis.

Treatment

The treatment of nasolacrimal tearing includes the use of topical antibiotic for a conjunctival infection, warm compresses, systemic antibiotics, nasal decongestants, and needle aspiration or an incision and drainage may be needed.

Globe Rupture

Globe rupture is a major ocular emergency that results from blunt or penetrating trauma, such as is caused by perforations with a sharp object. In order for a globe to rupture, there must be a perforation of the cornea and/or the sclera of the eye.

There are both anterior and posterior segment injuries that can occur. Anterior injuries affect the cornea, anterior chamber, iris and lens; posterior injuries can affect the sclera, retina and vitreous.

Signs and Symptoms

Some of the signs of globe rupture are decreased intraocular pressure, pigment under the conjunctiva, chemosis, peaked pupil, restricted eye movement, and vitreous hemorrhage. The pupil of the eye will assume a teardrop shape with the tip pointing towards the perforation. Patients with a ruptured globe may experience nausea and eye pain.

Treatment

When a globe rupture is suspected, avoid manipulating the eye; implanted objects should only be removed by an ophthalmologist. Instead, secure the foreign body and patch the other eye to decrease movement and prevent further damage. Aggressive pain management will help prevent/decrease the expulsion of intraocular contents. The patient should avoid any straining, bending over, lying in a flat position, coughing or gagging, and lifting any heavy objects.

Any surgical treatment that may be needed in the treatment of globe rupture(s) depends on the location, extent, and the type of foreign body, etc. The outcomes in terms of vision vary and they depend on the extent of the injury; children tend to have worse visual outcomes than adults do.

Ulcerations/Keratitis

Corneal ulcer or ulcerative keratitis is an inflammatory or infectious condition of the cornea. The noninfectious type of keratitis can be caused by a minor injury, such as wearing contact lenses too long. Infectious keratitis, on the other hand, can be caused by bacteria, viruses, fungi and parasites.

Signs and Symptoms

The signs and symptoms include redness of the eye, pain, excessive tearing, eye discharge, blurred vision, a decrease in vision, photophobia, a feeling of something in the eye, and difficulty opening the eyelid due to pain or discomfort.

Treatment

Treatment for noninfectious keratitis depends on the cause, but if it is due to a scratch or the extended wearing of contact lenses, treatment may include wearing a patch for 24 hours and topical medications.

Treatment for infectious keratitis depends on the cause. Antibacterial eye drops may be used for mild bacterial keratitis, and for moderate to severe cases, oral antibiotics may also be necessary; antifungal eye drops and oral antifungal medications may be prescribed for fungal keratitis; antiviral eye drops or oral antiviral medications may be effective for viral keratitis. Antibiotic eye drops may be effective in treating *acanthamoeba* keratitis but severe cases may require a corneal transplant.

Alzheimer's Disease/Dementia

Dementia is not a specific disease, but rather a group of symptoms that affect thinking and social abilities so severely that they interfere with the patient's everyday life and functioning. Unlike delirium, which can be treated and reversed, most cases of dementia are irreversible. Alzheimer's is the main cause of progressive dementia.

Signs and Symptoms

The signs and symptoms of dementia vary depending on the actual cause of the dementia. Some examples include hallucination, delusions, memory loss, agitation, paranoia, personality changes and problems performing usual activities. Nurses must modify care and communication as based on the patient's symptoms.

Treatment

The exact prevention of dementia is not known, but it has been shown that some things can lessen symptoms and slow down the progression of this disorder. Some recommendations for the patient include keeping an active mind, remaining physically and socially active, decreasing the blood pressure and healthy eating. Some helpful medications include memantine and cholinesterase inhibitors.

Multiple Sclerosis

Multiple Sclerosis (MS) is a progressive neurologic disease. It is believed to result from an autoimmune response to a viral infection, genetic susceptibility or an allergic reaction to an infection. Patients with MS have injury, destruction and malformation of the myelin sheaths that cover the nerves. These sheathes are destroyed in patches, known as plaques, along the axon. This destruction distorts the conduction of nerve impulses, and in some cases, it can cause the complete absence of impulse transmission. The neurons located in the optic nerve, cerebral and cerebellar areas, brainstem or spinal cord are usually affected by MS.

Signs and Symptoms

The signs and symptoms that a patient with MS experiences is dependent upon what area the disease affects. The most difficult symptom is chronic, extreme fatigue, which most MS sufferers experience. Other signs and symptoms include:

- Problems with vision, such as blurriness, haziness, color vision deficits, visual field deterioration and abnormal pupil reaction to light

- Alteration to the patient's mood, such as depression

- Lesions in the brainstem, which causes eye pain, diplopia, facial weakness, decreased sensations, vomiting, deafness, vertigo and nystagmus

- Cognitive dysfunction that can involve the patient's ability to concentrate, their short-term memory, word finding and panning

- Some other less common symptoms include extremity numbness, blindness, bladder problems and bowel problems.

It is difficult to diagnose MS, because it does not present uniformly. Tests include lumbar puncture, CT scan, evoked response, an MRI to detect plaques, cerebrospinal fluid analysis and positron emission tomography scanning.

Some of the complications associated with this disorder include difficulties performing the normal daily activities of life, level of independence, sexual function, mobility, airway clearance and the patient's overall ability to cope.

Treatment

Although there is no cure for MS, treatment aims to eliminate and decrease exacerbations and to increase remissions. Drug therapies include corticosteroids and glucocorticoids. Depression can be treated with antidepressants; muscle relaxants are used to treat spasms. For urinary problems, other medications can help.

Surgery may be indicated when the patient has extreme spasticity or deformity. Physical therapy and rehabilitation therapies are used depending on the patient's level of functioning. The ultimate goal of all treatments is to enable the patient to maintain their independence as long as possible, using assistive devices as indicated.

Myasthenia Gravis

Myasthenia gravis is a chronic, autoimmune neuromuscular disease. This disease affects the skeletal muscles of the body with fatigue and severe weakness. Antibodies destroy or block neuromuscular junction receptor sites, which results in a decreased number of acetylcholine receptors. The patient's muscular contractions are diminished even though there is a sufficient amount of acetylcholine.

Signs and Symptoms

Initially, the patient with myasthenia gravis will experience changes in their eye muscles, which present as diplopia or ptosis. Later, the patient will notice weaknesses to the facial, speech and mastication muscles, which can lead to the patients experiencing periods of dysarthria and dysphagia. Other symptoms include extreme fatigue, a smile that appears like a snarl or a grimace, changes in the voice, diminished vocalization, poor motor skills and a tendency for the head to roll into a forward position due the weakness in the neck muscles.

Some complications include increased risk for pneumonia due to weaknesses of the muscles of respiration, such as the diaphragm, that compromises gas exchange. Life-threatening emergencies, such as myasthenic crisis and cholinergic crisis, can occur.

Treatment

Anticholinesterases are the primary medications, and the most common of these are pyridostigmine (Mestinon). Prednisone, an immunosuppressive, and glucocorticoids are also used to improve muscular strength. If the prednisone is not effective, other medications such as azathioprine (Imuran) or cyclosporine can be combined with it. A thymectomy is another option for those patients less than 60 years of age who have dysplasia of the thymus gland.

Guillain-Barre Syndrome

Guillain-Barre syndrome is an acquired inflammatory condition that leads to peripheral nerve demyelination. The primary causative microorganism is *Campylobacter jejuni*.

Signs and Symptoms

Signs and symptoms can vary; however, some include bilateral ascending paralysis, sensory alterations like pain, decreased or absent deep tendon reflexes paresthesia, numbness, autonomic nervous system dysfunction as demonstrated with profuse diaphoresis, the lack of sweating, blood pressure and heart rate changes.

Treatment

Prompt diagnosis and treatment are essential to prevent respiratory failure and respiratory arrest. Diagnostic tests include electromyography (EMG), cerebrospinal fluid analysis, which will reveal increased protein levels in the presence of Guillain-Barre syndrome, and nerve conduction studies. Guillain-Barre syndrome is a life threatening condition with high morbidity and mortality rates. The ABCs are critical. Many patients need mechanical intervention for a prolonged period until the inflammatory process has ceased. Emergency department patients are typically hospitalized for an extended period, after which, extensive monitoring is required.

Temporal Arteritis

Temporal arteritis is damage and inflammation of the temporal artery, which supplies the brain with oxygenated blood. The artery becomes painful, tender, inflamed and swollen. The cause of temporal arteritis is not clear; however, it appears to be associated with a history of antibiotic use for an infection, a faulty immune response, and the presence of another autoimmune disorder.

Signs and Symptoms

The signs and symptoms of temporal arteritis are a throbbing, severe headache, anorexia, jaw pain, muscular aches, stiffness and pain, scalp tenderness, flu-like symptoms like fever and malaise, visual changes such as blurred or double vision, facial pain and hearing loss.

Treatment

After a temporal artery biopsy to establish diagnosis, the patient is treated with corticosteroids, supplemental vitamin D and calcium, aspirin in a low dose, and methotrexate, as indicated. The patient should avoid alcohol and tobacco.

Migraines

A migraine headache is a frequent cause of emergency department admissions. Although its cause is not definitive, it appears to be associated with a number of genetic and/or environmental factors such as hormone levels and gender. It appears that a migraine headache occurs when the cerebral cortex is overly excited and/or pain neurons are functioning abnormally. Migraine headaches are classified as a migraine without aura, or "common migraine", a migraine with aura, or "classic migraine", periodic childhood syndrome, a retinal migraine and chronic migraine.

Signs and Symptoms

The classic signs and symptoms of a migraine headache include a pulsating, severe headache that can last for hours, nausea, vomiting, and a sensitivity to sounds and light. The symptoms tend to worsen when the patient's activity level increases. Some patients also experience an aura, which can include motor, language, visual, and language-related disturbances.

Treatment

Treatment includes analgesics such as acetaminophen or ibuprofen, antiemetics, metoclopramide, intranasal lidocaine, and ergotamines or triptan medications if simple analgesic therapy does not relieve the symptoms. Alternative therapies can include acupuncture, neuro-stimulation, acupressure, chiropractic, magnesium vitamin B12, biofeedback and relaxation techniques.

Increased Intracranial Pressure (ICP)

Normal intracranial pressure (ICP) ranges from 5 to 15 mmHg. Increased ICP occurs when the volume of the cranial cavity increases, as can occur with a closed head trauma, a cerebral infarction, a subdural or epidural hematoma, infection and the presence of a cerebral tumor. Brain herniation and death occurs when intracranial pressure increases without successful treatment.

Signs and Symptoms

Some of the commonly occurring signs and symptoms include Cushing's and Cheyne-Stokes respirations. Cushing's reflex indicates that brainstem ischemia is present; it is characterized by bradycardia, a widening pulse pressure and hypertension.

Treatment

The goal of treatment is the preservation of life and the prevention of permanent disorders. Some of the medications used include corticosteroids to reduce edema, intravenous osmotic diuretics like mannitol to remove fluid, and anticonvulsant medications to prevent seizures. A barbiturate coma is sometimes induced to lower the metabolic demands of the brain and to prevent further brain damage. Additionally, artificial ventilation is often needed; surgical interventions are sometimes indicated to eliminate the cause of the ICP.

Bacterial Meningitis

Meningitis is an infection of the meninges that encircle the brain and the spinal cord. This infection can also invade the arachnoid mater, the pia mater and the subarachnoid space. The two classifications of meningitis are viral and bacterial. Meningitis is an infectious disease and a life threatening neurological emergency. Significant mortality and morbidity are associated with bacterial meningitis.

Neisseria meningitides, Hemophilus influenzae and *Streptococcus pneumoniae* are the most common bacterial agents that cause meningitis. Other less common pathogens include *listeria monocytogenes, E. coli* and *staphylococcus aureus*.

Signs and Symptoms

Bacterial symptoms include generalized back, abdominal or limb pain, chills, fever, photophobia, petechial rash, tachycardia, neck stiffness, severe headache, vomiting, nausea, focal neurological deficits, seizures, and altered level of consciousness. A positive Brudzinski's sign and Kernig's sign indicate the presence of meningitis.

Treatment

Early antibiotic therapy is indicated. Third-generation cephalosporins and benzylpenicillin are most often used. In conjunction with antibiotics, corticosteroids are common. Other interventions include seizure management, analgesia, hydration, the constant use of the ABCs and monitoring the patient's level of consciousness.

Viral Meningitis

Viral meningitis is the most common form. Viral meningitis can be caused by herpes simplex 2, Epstein-Barr, HIV, varicella zoster, Coxsackie, mumps and enterovirus.

Signs and Symptoms

Viral meningitis signs and symptoms are highly similar to those associated with bacterial meningitis; however, they are usually less severe because viral meningitis is typically limited to the meninges only. Analysis of cerebrospinal fluid will reveal normal glucose content, moderate increases in protein and increased lymphocytes.

Treatment

Acute viral meningitis is often self-limiting; interventions aim to treat the associated symptoms. Antiviral agents, such as acyclovir, are often indicated when the patient is affected with HSV-2 viral meningitis.

Seizure Disorders

Seizures occur due to abnormal electrical activity in the brain. An epileptic seizure disorder, more commonly known as epilepsy, is a disorder in which a person has two or more unprovoked seizures. This brain disorder's cause is often unknown. Symptomatic epilepsy can be caused by strokes, tumors or malformations.

Seizures caused by temporary disorders or stressors are called non-epileptic seizures. Some of the causes are things like severe hypoglycemia, central nervous system infections, drug use or withdrawal, cardiovascular disorders and metabolic disorders.

Seizures that occur due to a known cause, such as a stroke or brain tumor, are known as symptomatic seizures. These types of seizures are common mostly among the neonatal and elderly age groups.

Generalized seizures impair motor function throughout the seizure and the patient will usually become unconscious. The different types of generalized seizures include infantile spasms, which affect young children less than five years of age, juvenile myoclonic epilepsy, typical absence seizures, atypical absence seizures, atonic seizures, tonic seizures, tonic clonic seizures, myoclonic seizures, febrile seizures, and status epilepticus.

Infantile spasms result from developmental defects; typical absence seizures are accompanied by a very brief loss of consciousness, no convulsions and the patient simply stops their current activity with no recollection that they have even had a seizure. These types of seizures are most common among children and are they are genetically inherited. Atypical absence seizures usually occur in patients that have Lennox-Gastaut syndrome, which is a severe form of epilepsy. These seizures also occur among young children; they have a longer duration, lower pronounced loss of consciousness and more dramatic jerking than a typical absence seizure. Atonic seizures also present in children as part of Lennox-Gastaut syndrome. Children experiencing these types of seizures will fall to the ground and experienced short-lived, though complete, loss of consciousness and muscle control.

Tonic seizures occur usually in children while they are asleep. This type of seizures last about ten to fifteen seconds. They can be generalized either primarily or secondarily. In the primarily generalized form, the patient calls out, falls and loses consciousness. The muscles of the head, extremities, and legs then rapidly begin contracting and relaxing. There is also occasional tongue biting, frothing of the mouth, and urinary and fecal incontinence. The secondary forms of these seizures start with a complex partial or simple partial seizure.

Myoclonic seizures are short-lived seizures. Single limbs, several limbs or the trunk can begin quick jerking motions during these seizures, which don't usually involve loss of consciousness unless they evolve into generalized tonic clonic seizures. Juvenile myoclonic epilepsy is an epilepsy syndrome that normally presents in adolescents and can manifest with myoclonic, tonic clonic and absence seizures.

Febrile seizures are considered a type of provoked seizure, which occur when the patient has a fever but has no intracranial infection. The two types are benign and complicated. With benign type, the patient experiences a short, solitary and generalized seizure that is tonic-clonic in appearance. With the complicated form, seizures can last more than fifteen minutes or recur two or more times in 24 hours.

Status epilepticus is a life-threatening condition. This condition is characterized by unrelenting, persistent seizure activity without regaining consciousness between the seizures. It is a medical emergency.

A partial seizure, also referred to as a focal seizure, is subcategorized as simple partial seizures, epilepsia partialis continua, which is rare, and complex partial seizures. During a simple partial seizure, the patient is conscious, but experiences motor, sensory or psychomotor symptoms. An Epilepsia partialis continuum entails focal motor seizures involving the hand, arm or one side of the face. Complex partial seizures are often accompanied by a patient trance or stare; the person remains conscious during the seizure, but is somewhat impaired. Motor system alterations with things like lip smacking, hand jerking, and uncontrollable leg movements occur.

Signs and Symptoms:

The majority of seizures tend to last between thirty seconds to two minutes. Any seizure lasting for more than five minutes is considered an emergency. If a victim has several seizures and/or does not regain consciousness, it is an emergency.

There are a wide variety of signs and symptoms associated with seizure activity. Some of the most common signs and symptoms include staring, loss of bladder control, loss of bowel control, confusion, loss of consciousness, repeated jerking of the limb(s), convulsions, lip smacking, hand rubbing, perceiving an odd smell, sound or taste, picking at clothes, drowsiness, altered responsiveness, and visual spots.

Treatment

Treatments are determined on a case-by-case manner; the ultimate goal is to address the cause of the seizure(s). There are several different types of medications available for the treatment of seizure disorders including Ativan, Cerebyx, Dilantin, Luminal, Depakote, and Topamax; surgery is indicated when the patient is not responding to medications and the cerebral area that is affected is small and localized.

Patients who are diagnosed with seizure disorders should be encouraged to wear a medical alert bracelet, get adequate rest and avoid all possible seizure triggers.

Shunt Dysfunctions

Brain shunts are often used to decrease intracranial pressure secondary to hydrocephalus. These divert fluid from the brain to other bodily parts for absorption. Brain shunt dysfunctions are a life-threatening medical emergency.

There are several types of shunts, including

- Ventriculo-peritoneal shunts, which drain the brain's ventricle into the abdominal cavity

- Ventriculo-pleural shunts, which move the fluid into the pleural space surrounding the lung

- Ventriculo-atrial shunts that move fluid from the brain to the right atrium of the heart

Some shunts are programmable to control the amount of fluid drained; others have fixed pressure that drains at a set rate. Shunt malfunction and failure is life threatening and can occur secondary to an obstruction, disconnection, migration, fracture, ascites, abdominal pseudo-cyst, infections, and even constipation. These can be classified as over-draining and under-draining dysfunctions.

Signs and Symptoms

Over-draining dysfunctions tear blood vessels and collapse ventricles. Symptoms include headache, hemorrhage secondary to subdural hematoma and slit ventricle syndrome. Under-draining dysfunctions occur when the cerebrospinal fluid does not adequately drain and the signs and symptoms of hydrocephalus return, in addition to infections, which are marked by a fever, sore shoulder and neck muscles, as well as tenderness and pain along the tract of the shunt. Shunt obstructions lead to under-draining dysfunctions. The signs and symptoms of hydrocephalus include nausea, vomiting, papilledema, and headache, among others.

Treatment

Immediate treatment includes relief of intracranial pressure and correction of existing complications. Later treatments include repair and/or placement of another shunt as indicated. Infections, a major and common complication of brain shunts, are aggressively treated according to the causative pathogen.

Spinal Cord Injuries

Spinal cord injuries are frequently encountered in the emergency department. According to the American Spinal Injury Association's ASIA scale, these are classified from Grades A to E according to motor and sensory deficits. Spinal cord injuries are also categorized as tetraplegia and paraplegia injuries. Tetraplegia is the loss or impairment of sensory and/or motor function originating at the cervical portion of the spinal cord. This type of injury causes absent or diminished functioning of the trunk, pelvic organs arms and legs. Paraplegia, on the other hand, is the loss or diminished functioning of sensory and/or motor function from the thoracic, lumbar or sacral portion of the spinal cord. This type of injury causes impaired functioning of the pelvic organs, trunk, and legs without any arm involvement.

Spinal cord injuries are also categorized according to the type of force exerted to produce it. These forces include flexion, extension, compression and rotation.

Flexion motion injuries, or burst fractures, most commonly occur with a car accident when the neck is hyper-flexed as the victim's chin is forced into the chest; it dislocates the spine and ruptures posterior ligaments. Extension injuries, referred to as hangman's fractures, occur when the head is tossed backwards; it fractures the posterior aspects of the vertebral body and ruptures the anterior ligament.

Compression injuries, or axial load injuries, can result from a dive into shallow water or a serious fall; the vertebral bodies become compressed and wedged and bone shards pierce the spinal cord. Rotational injuries can occur as the result of a variety of injuries and they are the most unstable of all flexion rotation injuries; these injuries damage the entire ligamentous structure.

All spinal cord injuries, except those that result from a gunshot or stabbing wound, are non-penetrating. Penetrating spinal cord injuries are serious and unstable.

Signs and Symptoms

The signs and symptoms of spinal cord injuries vary according to the type and extent of the injury. Other signs of spinal cord injuries include the compromise of the ABCs, impaired vital lung capacity, aspiration, hypoxia, impaired gas exchange and diminished respiratory muscle function, all of which can be fatal if untreated.

Other possible signs and symptoms include pain, nausea, vomiting, impaired urinary function, paralytic ileus, and hypothermia, in addition to motor and sensory impairments including paralysis. After the most severe and life-threatening conditions are treated, further assessments are done as the nurse ensures that no flexion, extension or rotation of the patient's spine occurs. Log-rolling and careful clothing removal ensures spine stability.

Some of the commonly occurring complications of spinal cord injury include:

- Neurogenic shock, most often the result of a spinal cord injury at or below the T6 level, can lead to life threatening complications like massive vasodilation, diminished venous return, alterations of tissue perfusion and decreased cardiac output. Neurogenic shock is characterized by hypotension, as the result of peripheral vasodilation, the loss of sweating below the injury, hypothermia, as the result of impaired sympathetic nervous system functioning, altered hypothalamus functioning, hypotension and bradycardia.

- Spinal shock, which can persist for weeks after a cervical or upper thoracic spinal cord injury, can lead to a loss of functioning below the injury level, and other symptoms like flaccid paralysis of the bowel and bladder, and priapism.

- Poikilothermia, the body's loss of ability to control and regulate body temperature, is most commonly associated with injuries at and above T6. It is signaled with sweating and shivering, so it is important that body temperature is monitored and environmental temperature is controlled.

- Autonomic dysreflexia, a life-threatening condition, occurs among patients with a spinal cord injury at or above T6. Autonomic dysreflexia is precipitated with bowel or bladder distention renal stones, tight clothing, a urinary tract infection, fractures, and hemorrhoids. Some of the signs and symptoms of autonomic dysreflexia are high blood pressure, headache, paleness, pallor, shortness of breath, anxiety, blurry vision and compensatory bradycardia.

Treatment includes the identification and elimination of the precipitating cause and the use of nitrates or nifedipine.

Treatment

The spine is kept in neutral alignment and immobilized at all times with the exception of when the airway has to be opened to sustain life. A Kendrick Extrication Device (KED), used in addition to a cervical collar, sandbags or commercially available head restraints, are used to immobilize a patient's head, neck and spine in the normal anatomical, or neutral, position. Severe to moderate pain is treated with morphine or fentanyl. Anticonvulsants, tricyclic antidepressants, antiemetics and a nasogastric tube for distention, the prevention of a paralytic ileus, nausea and vomiting, as well as intubation and mechanical intervention are often indicated.

Prophylactic anticoagulant therapy with low-molecular-weight heparin or low-dose heparin, compression stockings and intermittent sequential calf-compression devices are used to prevent deep vein thrombosis.

A urinary catheter is used to treat a contractile neuropathic bladder and to ensure adequate urinary output. Intake and output are monitored and documented.

Spinal Cord Compression

Spinal cord compression is an emergency that can lead to irreversible paraplegia.

Risk factors for spinal cord compression are pressure from expanding tumors, such as those of the lung or prostate. It is associated with lymphoma or metastatic disease.

Signs and Symptoms

Back pain, numbness, parenthesis, weakness, coldness of the leg, leg pain, bladder and bowel dysfunction, and paralysis can occur.

Treatment

Treatment for spinal cord compression can be rendered with either radiation or a surgical intervention.

Stroke: Ischemic and Hemorrhagic

Strokes are a major neurological event that can lead to death and permanent disability. They are classified according to cause - ischemia or hemorrhage.

Ischemic Stroke

Simply stated, ischemic strokes occur when essential blood and oxygen supply to the brain is adversely affected. These strokes can result from emboli, thrombi and hypoperfusion, which is the rarest of all stroke causes. Cardiac arrhythmias are the most common cause of hypoperfusion strokes.

Embolic strokes occur when a blood vessel is occluded with a clot that has traveled to the brain from another part of the body including from the major vessels of the heart. Cardiogenic emboli most often occur as the result of atrial fibrillation and valve disease; however, they can also result from a septic embolus, a fat embolus and as the result of illicit intravenous drug abuse.

Thrombosis secondary to clot formation is one of the most common causes of stroke. Arthrosclerosis, some infectious diseases, polycythemia and vasculitis are some of the risk factors associated with this type of ischemic stroke.

Hemorrhagic Stroke

Hemorrhagic strokes are mostly caused by hypertension, but other causes can include head trauma, brain tumors, a ruptured aneurysm, and vascular malformations. Decreased perfusion and increased intracranial pressure associated with this type of stroke lead to cerebral injury and damage.

Signs and Symptoms

The signs and symptoms of stroke vary according to the type of stroke and the area of the brain that is adversely affected. When anterior circulation is adversely affected, the signs and symptoms include sensory and motor facial and lower extremity deficits, dysphagia, visual alterations, mathematical and writing difficulties, urinary deficits, personality changes and left-sided unilateral neglect.

Posterior circulation disruptions lead to ataxia, diplopia, vertigo, nystagmus, visual disturbances, and bilateral or unilateral sensory and motor deficits. Strokes affecting the brainstem typically present with altered level of consciousness and severe respiratory compromise, including a respiratory arrest.

Treatment

Strokes are considered an emergency and should be treated as such. Prompt diagnosis, treatment and referral are essential to ensure the best patient outcomes, to prevent complications and to prevent permanent deformity and dysfunction.

The prevention of complications within the first twenty-four to forty-eight hours is essential to decrease stroke-related mortality and disability. For example, thrombolytic medications should be administered in a timely and prompt manner within three to four and a half hours after the onset of symptoms. Other treatment interventions, as indicated by the cause, type of stroke, and site of the stroke include:

- Patients must have adequate ventilation, oxygenation and cerebral perfusion. Airway support with endotracheal intubation and mechanical ventilation may be indicated. Their ABCs require constant monitoring.

- Patients who are hypoxic with a peripheral oxygen saturation of less than 92-95% need supplemental oxygen.

- Hypotension and dehydration should be treated cautiously with intravenous fluids and vasopressors as needed. Fluid overload must be avoided.

- Medications to prevent venous thrombosis are administered prophylactically.

- Referrals for follow-up care include physiotherapy, speech therapy and dietary management, as indicated by the patient's condition. Within the first twenty-four to forty-eight hours, the patient should be assessed for problems relating to swallowing, nutrition, speech, and mobility.

The Treatment of Ischemic Stroke

Aspirin is beneficial to reducing mortality and recurrent stroke. Other anticoagulants, including low-molecular-weight heparin, are not used. Anticonvulsant agents, like phenytoin, are indicated in the presence of seizures.

The Treatment of Hemorrhagic Stroke

Intracerebral hemorrhage management depends on the cause, location, and the patient's condition, including the presence of any neurological deficits. Cerebral edema and increased intracranial pressure have to be monitored and treated.

Transient Ischemic Attack

Transient ischemic attacks (TIA) closely mimic a stroke but they typically last only a short period and do not cause permanent disability. However, TIAs are a serious warning sign of impending stroke.

Signs and Symptoms

The signs and symptoms of a transient ischemic attack can be classified as anterior and posterior circulation syndromes. Posterior circulation transient ischemic attacks are associated with ataxia, hemiparesis, dysphagia, and other signs and symptoms; anterior circulation syndromes are characterized by hemiparesis, visual disturbances, aphasia, unilateral sensory losses, and other signs and symptoms. Other common signs of a TIA include sudden hypertension, unconsciousness, confusion, arm and/or leg numbness and tingling, loss of balance, muscular weakness, dizziness, sudden fatigue, temporary memory loss, personality changes and speech changes.

Treatment

The primary focus of care is the identification and treatment of an underlying cause to prevent a possibly permanently disabling stroke. Cerebral perfusion is maintained with supplemental oxygen and the avoidance of antihypertensive medications.

Antiplatelet medications, liked ticlodipine, aspirin-dipyridamole and clopidogrel, are useful for the prevention of other TIAs and stroke. A carotid endarterectomy may be indicated for those at risk.

Treatments will also help to prevent strokes in the future. Common plans of action include the control of diabetes, hypertension, hyperlipidemia and quitting smoking. Lifestyle changes, such as diet and exercise, also help prevent future strokes.

Most uncomplicated patients can be discharged to the home from the ER for follow-up care in the community; however, those at high risk for stroke may require acute care and hospitalization until they are stable.

Traumatic Head and Brain Injuries

Traumatic brain injuries impact the whole patient, physically, psychologically and socially. It can lead to death, permanent and irreversible brain damage, as well as cognitive losses. There are several types of physiological injuries that can occur at the moment of trauma, including damage to the blood vessels, increased intracranial pressure, contusions, diffuse axonal shearing which is the stretching, cutting and tearing of the neurons' axons, and cellular death. When intracranial pressure gets too high, it can lead to brain herniation and death may occur.

The signs and symptoms can include pain, changes in the patient's level of consciousness, cognitive changes, hypocapnia (increased levels of carbon dioxide in the blood) hypotension, hypoxia and acidosis.

Treatment

Decreasing intracranial pressure is a patient care priority. Oxygenation, ventilation, circulating volume replacement and blood pressure maintenance are some of the priorities of care.

Orthopedic Emergencies

Amputation

Traumatic amputation is a partial or complete removal of an extremity as the result of a traumatic event or accident. Traumatic amputation often negatively impacts on the physical and psychological wellbeing of the patient as well as their family.

Traumatic amputations are classified according to the nature of the cause. Crush amputations lead to soft tissue and vascular damage, avulsion amputations tear and/or stretch the limb until it separates, and guillotine amputations have a well-defined perimeter that causes damage to vessels, tissue and nerves. Occupational risks for amputation are associated with jobs that use heavy equipment.

Signs and Symptoms

The signs and symptoms include the obvious loss of part or an entire limb or digit. This loss is accompanied by bleeding, pain and severe anxiety.

Treatment

The goal of emergency interventions in the emergency department aims to maintain the limb and its functioning and to ensure the ABCs, since traumatic amputations are often associated with patients who present with severe blood loss and multiple traumas. Care of the amputated part includes keeping it dry and cool after it is cleaned with sterile saline and placed in a sealed plastic bag in ice. Freezing can lead to tissue necrosis.

A tetanus vaccine and antibiotics prevent infection; a surgical reattachment of the bodily part is performed if possible. Soft tissue that is devascularized, delayed surgical correction and severe crush injuries are often not re-implanted successfully. Other priority interventions include the treatment of toxicity from deviated tissue (rhabdomyolysis), infection, acidosis, hypothermia, and bleeding.

Compartment Syndrome

Compartment syndrome results from increased pressure within an anatomical area that impairs the circulation and viability of the tissues. Compartment syndrome can occur with anything restrictive, including a cast after a fracture that becomes tight as the result of swelling. Potassium is released from damaged cells and protein breakdown occurs. These changes place the patient at risk for shock, renal failure, and acidosis as the intravascular fluid moves into the third, or interstitial, spaces. The fascia becomes tighter; tissue ischemia and necrosis occur within about six hours when this buildup of fluid and the pressure are not relieved. In severe cases, myoglobinuria can lead to sepsis, metabolic acidosis, renal failure and hyperkalemia. Compartment syndrome is a limb and life-threatening emergency

Signs and Symptoms

The earliest sign of compartment syndrome is pain not alleviated by elevation and analgesics. This ischemic pain is described by patients as throbbing, deep and/or burning, and it often worsens with limb movement. Paresthesia is also an early sign of compartment syndrome; it results from direct pressure on the nerves. The patient typically reports numbness, feelings of pressure, tingling or burning.

Hypoesthesia, another neurological complication of compartment syndrome, occurs when the sensory nerves lose sensitivity. Signs and symptoms of hypoesthesia include muscular weakness and paralysis (late symptoms of untreated compartmental syndrome), skin pallor and coolness to the touch, and an inability to detect a pulse.

Treatment

The treatment aims to immediately reduce and eliminate any pressure on the tissue, nerves and circulatory system so the bodily part and its full functioning can be restored. Blood flow must be restored in order to achieve this treatment goal. Cast removal is often necessary. At times, a surgical intervention, such as a fasciotomy or epimysiotomy, is indicated when the pressure is severely higher than the normal range from 1 to 10 mm HG. Nurses must monitor the patient's pressures using a compartment pressure monitor, pulses, level of pain, and neurovascular status on an hourly basis until stabilized. The limb, or body part, should also be elevated unless contraindicated.

Bivalve casts are preferred over closed casts for extremity fracture immobilization because they allow room for swelling and, therefore, can successfully prevent compartment syndrome.

Other Traumatic Injuries

Injury	Description	Signs and Symptoms	Treatment
Abrasions	A skin friction wound that involves one or more layers of the epidermis to be removed	Pain, redness and minor bleeding	Wound irrigation/debridement. Abrasions are kept moist to aid healing; Non-adherent, sterile dressing placed over wound.
Avulsions	Avulsions are the traumatic tearing away and loss of the epidermis and dermis	Pain, bleeding and skin integrity alterations	Wound irrigation/debridement; approximation of wound edges is not possible; Severe injuries may require skin grafting
Contusions	Contusions from blunt trauma cause rupture of blood vessels and bleeding into local tissues; can be superficial or deep	Discomfort and pain Ecchymosis	NSAIDs for pain; RICE (rest, ice, compression and elevation) Light stretching exercises may be indicated
Hematomas	Results from blunt trauma; Patients taking anticoagulants or with coagulopathy are at greatest risk.	Swelling and pain Bruising	Compression, elevation and ice to promote vasoconstriction and decrease of blood flow Sutures for ruptured vessels Larger hematomas can be drained or evacuated
Lacerations	The skin is torn or cut and separated without other tissue loss	Pain and bleeding	Irrigation/debridement; sutures may be necessary for lacerations that are deep/ over moving joints; wound closure strips for superficial lacerations; 48 hours after closure non-adherent dressing should be applied until epithelial bridging occurs
Puncture wounds	Caused by penetration of skin by sharp object; often occurs on the feet; Increased risk of infection; Punctures close	Bleeding and pain	Cleansing and a sterile dressing for protection against infection Wounds are not be sutured closed, so that any debris can exit the wound Antibiotics, as indicated

	rapidly so cleaning deepest part of wound base is essential		
Foreign bodies	Foreign material can be left by any wound caused by a foreign object	Inflammatory processes greater when material produces toxins; Swelling; Granuloma	Removal is attempted
Bite wounds	Can be caused by animals or humans These puncture wounds can penetrate underlying structures, such as tendons, muscle, bone, joints, and ligaments	Pain and bleeding	All bites are considered contaminated with the risk of infection Copious irrigation and debridement Delayed closure in order to prevent deep infection, although facial wounds may have immediate closure for cosmetic appearances Antibiotics A cosmetic surgery referral is made as indicted
Oral and Lip Injuries	Occur with a blow to the face or a fall	Profuse bleeding and pain; broken or missing teeth, bite malocclusion or trismus	Minor wounds do not require closure, but full thickness wounds do, including large tongue lacerations; surface lip lacerations may require cosmetic closure; Patient education should include need for saline oral washes 6x/day especially after meals and only soft foods

Costochondritis

Costochondritis is an inflammation of the sternum at the costosternal junction. It is also known as chest wall pain, costosternal syndrome, and costosternal chondrodynia.

Signs and Symptoms

The pain mimics that of a heart attack or other heart conditions. When accompanied by swelling, it is known as Tietze syndrome. Pain and tenderness worsens when the patient takes deep breaths and coughs.

Treatment

Treatment includes over-the-counter pain relievers, and if they are not enough NSAIDs, narcotics, anti-seizure drugs, such as gabapentin, or tricyclic antidepressants, such as amitriptyline, may be prescribed. Physical therapy with stretching and the use of a TENS may be helpful. If other treatments don't work, then an anesthetic, numbing medication or a corticosteroid may be injected directly into the painful joint.

Fractures

Fractures result from a traumatic impact or some undue pressure on the bone that cannot be sustained without damage to the bone itself. Risk factors associated with fractures include age, bone size, bone density, neoplastic disease, a poor physical condition, and hazardous occupations and avocations. Many fractures occur as the result of an accident or trauma; however, some may also occur as bone stressors, as occurs among athletes. Fractures are classified in many ways, as below.

- An incomplete fracture where only a part of the bone is affected

- A complete fracture where the entire cross section of the bone is fractured

- A pathological fracture which results from weakened bones as a complication of a disease process rather than trauma or stress

- Unstable fractures which are displaced and require reduction

- Stable fractures which are not displaced so reduction is not necessary

- Open fractures, or compound fractures, break through the skin and soft tissue in the surrounding area

- Closed fractures, also referred to as a simple fractures, do not penetrate the skin. The skin remains intact.

Fractures are also described in terms of their pattern. The patterns associated with skeletal fractures are:

- Transverse fractures that go straight across the bone

- Spiral fractures that twist and turns around the bone

- Oblique fractures that cut across the bone at an angle

- Comminuted fractures which involve bone splinters and fragments

- Impacted fractures that lead to a part of the bone being impacted or wedged into another bone

- Compression fractures, which involve the collapse of the bone

- Greenstick fractures, which only affect one side of the bone

- Avulsion fractures that entail a bone fragment, which pulls off the bone at the tendon or ligament

- Depressed fractures, when bone fragments are driven inward

Signs and Symptoms

Some examples of the signs and symptoms of fractures are deformity, bruising at the site, swelling and tenderness, pain at the site, loss of function, a possible grating sensation and paresthesia.

Altered neurovascular status is signaled with progressive, uncontrollable pain, diminished capillary refill, paresthesia, loss of active motion, and diminished distal pulses with pallor

Treatment

All skeletal injuries can lead to serious neurological and vascular changes because of the fact that bones are proximate to, and surrounded by, circulatory vessels, peripheral sensory nerves and motor nerves.

Healing and the prevention of deformity are the goals of treatment. Fractures are immobilized with a splint in order to prevent further injury. Open wounds related to a compound open fracture and/or another traumatic injury are protected with a moist sterile dressing. Proper bodily alignment is ensured throughout care and treatment. Plaster casts, traction and other forms of immobilization, when indicated, must be applied with care and caution. Pain is managed with immobilization, elevation of the affect limb, the application of cool packs and analgesic medications.

Pelvic and Hip Fractures

Pelvic fractures can also be classified as lateral compression, anteroposterior, vertical shear and combined pelvic fractures.

Lateral compression pelvic fractures

These fractures occur as the result of a force or impact to the side of the pelvis. Minor lateral compression pelvic fractures are treated with bed rest; major lateral compression pelvic fractures are treated with an open reduction and internal fixation, and bed rest.

Anteroposterior compression fractures

An impact to the anterior aspect of the pelvis causes this type of pelvic fracture. It can lead to severe iliac vessel hemorrhage and death without treatment. When the symphysis pubis and innominate bones separate more than 2 cm, it is considered unstable.

Vertical shear pelvic fractures

These fractures commonly occur from a fall. This trauma can lead to serious neurological damage and it is usually treated with stabilization using traction, internal fixation or internal fixation depending on the particular injury.

Combined fractures of the pelvis

Combined pelvic fractures are usually unstable; they are defined as those pelvic fractures that occur as a combination of several mechanisms and several fracture patterns. The elderly population is at greatest risk for proximal femur and femoral neck fractures, although it can occur among younger populations. These fractures are possibly the most frequently encountered skeletal injury in emergency departments. The morbidity and mortality rates associated with this trauma injury are high, and hip fractures among the younger population are associated with higher rates of necrosis than those found among the elderly.

Signs and Symptoms

Patients who present with this type of injury usually cannot straighten or rotate the leg on the affected side, experience pain when the leg is manipulated. The patient most often presents with their leg externally rotated.

Treatment

The stabilization of the pelvis is necessary to reduce the risk of clot formation, hemodynamic instability, bleeding and pain. This stabilization is accomplished with a pelvic binder, a C clamp or an external fixator. Pain management medications are used and a wedge is placed between the patient's knees for immobilization.

Necrotizing Fasciitis

Necrotizing fasciitis is also referred to as gas gangrene, Fournier gangrene, streptococcus hemolytic gangrene and "flesh eating" bacteria. It can develop quickly after trauma and affects underlying subcutaneous tissue and fascia. Gram-negative microorganisms, often in combination with anaerobic bacteria, are often the offending pathogens, especially tissue hypoxia. Infected wounds are prone to it.

Signs and Symptoms

Erythema, swelling, pain, fever and chills are some of the signs and symptoms of necrotizing fasciitis. Skin changes such as bullae, skin ulceration, necrotic black scabs, and wound drainage occurs. Sepsis and death can also occur.

Treatment

The treatment of necrotizing fasciitis includes aggressive antibiotic treatment, debriding the wound and supportive treatments such as fluids and hyperbaric oxygen therapy. Most, if not all, patients with necrotizing fasciitis are hospitalized; the associated morbidity and mortality rates are high.

Joint Effusion

A joint effusion is the collection of increased intra-articular fluid in a joint. The knee is most often affected by joint effusion. It can occur from infections, trauma, tumors, cysts, overuse, obesity, vigorous exercise and sports, inflammation and some conditions like osteoarthritis, rheumatoid arthritis, gout, and bursitis.

Signs and Symptoms

The signs and symptoms include pain, swelling, and joint stiffness.

Treatment

Treatments are based on the identification and correction of the underlying cause(s) in addition to analgesics, joint rest, and the application of cold and joint aspiration, as indicated.

Low Back Pain

Most people experience low back pain at least once in their lives; in fact, back pain is the most common reason for visits to the doctor and missed days of work.

Signs and Symptoms

Signs and symptoms include muscular aches, shooting or stabbing pain, limited flexibility and range of motion and the inability to stand up straight.

Treatment

Treatment in most cases just requires over the counter pain relievers and anti-inflammatory medications, rest and restriction to light activity. In some severe cases, narcotics, such as codeine or hydrocodone, low doses of some tricyclic antidepressants, such as amitriptyline, and a referral to a pain management specialist are indicated. Physical therapy and exercise can also help to ease the pain. In other cases, an injection of cortisone into the epidural space can help to relieve the pain for up to a few months. Surgery is rarely necessary.

Osteomyelitis

Osteomyelitis is a very serious bone infection that can lead to tetanus, necrotizing fasciitis, septicemia, permanent damage, deformity and even death when left untreated. The population at greatest risk is those who have recently had a compound bone fracture that has disrupted the integrity of the skin, but those who have had an infection in another part of the body or after orthopedic surgery, particularly when rods and plates are used, are also at risk.

Other risk factors include hemodialysis, diabetes, a splenectomy, the use of illicit drugs and a poor blood supply. These infections are most commonly caused by the *staphylococcus aureus* pathogen but they can also occur as the result of fungi and other microorganisms.

Signs and Symptoms

The signs of infection, bone pain, lower extremity swelling, malaise and local redness, swelling and heat over the affected area.

Treatment

The goal of treatment is to resolve the infection with antibiotics and to prevent damage to surrounding areas. Irrigation and drainage, a surgical debridement and the removal of any orthopedic devices and prostheses, such as plates and rods is indicated when they are the cause of this serious bone infection.

Other Trauma

Achilles tendon injuries most commonly occur among athletes. Most are caused by tendonitis, and these injuries can be relatively minor. Some can be quite severe, as occurs when the tendon is completely or partially torn or ruptured. The risk factors associated with Achilles tendon injuries are athletic overuse, wearing high-heeled shoes, a failure to perform stretching before vigorous exercise, muscles and/or tendons that are abnormally tight, and anatomical abnormalities such as "flat feet".

Signs and Symptoms

Pain, tenderness, stiffness, swelling, trouble flexing the foot and hearing a snap at the time of the injury are the signs and symptoms.

Treatment

Treatment includes ice to reduce the pain and swelling, rest, leg compression with an elastic bandage, leg elevation, the use of a heel lift, stretching exercises and the use of NSAIDs to relieve pain and decrease swelling and inflammation.

Blast Injuries

Nurses working in the emergency department receive blast injury survivors when there is a major external disaster such as a chemical plant explosion or an act of terrorism. Blast waves transport objects including debris, human bodies, bodily parts, and the contents of the explosive device, such as nails.

Blast injuries are classified as primary, secondary and tertiary blast injuries. Primary injuries are the result of the blast waves' pressure and they affect the gas filled bodily organs. Secondary blast injuries result from flying debris and projectiles of all sorts; these penetrating blast injuries affect soft tissue. In contrast, tertiary blast injuries are typically blunt force trauma injuries that occur when victims are tossed about with the force of the blast. Miscellaneous blast injuries can include things like crush injuries, burns, inhalation injures and toxic blast injuries.

Signs and Symptoms

The signs and symptoms of primary blast injuries include sheared, disintegrated, stretched and compressed tissue as well as torn and lacerated internal organs. Gas-filled organs, including the bowels, ears, lungs and bowels, can be severely compromised with ischemia, rupture and hemorrhage.

The signs and symptoms of fragmentation blast injuries include a "peppered" skin appearance where fragments have entered, vascular lacerations and tearing and a number of other complications should as head injuries, hemorrhage, and a wide variety of other possibly life threatening side effects.

Treatment

The treatments vary according to the type of the injury, the extent of the injury and the medical status of the patient. First, and most importantly, the ABCs and other life threatening conditions are treated, as necessary. Other more general treatments include antibiotics, a tetanus vaccine, the treatment and correction of hemorrhage, surgery to remove foreign bodies when this can be safely done, wound cleansing, suturing, fracture care and management, incision and drainage, organ repair, major vessel ligation, and a guillotine amputation of the limb(s) when necessary.

Sprains

A sprain is a musculoskeletal minor injury that stretches or tears a ligament. Sprains can occur as the result of a fall, abnormal twisting, and blunt force trauma. These injuries most often affect the ankle or fingers used to break a fall.

Signs and Symptoms

The signs and symptoms of a sprain include bruising, poor joint movement, swelling and pain. Some patients may report that they heard a popping noise at the time of the injury.

Strains

A strain is a musculoskeletal minor injury that stretches or tears a tendon. Many people refer to strains as a "pulled muscle". Some strains are caused by overuse, trauma and using a muscle in an abnormal manner.

Signs and Symptoms

Signs and symptoms are pain, swelling, loss of limb function, and bruising.

Treatment of Strains and Sprains

Some of the treatments used for strains and sprains include the application of cold every hour for about 15 minutes, rest, elevation and over-the-counter anti-inflammatory and pain medications as needed.

Abrasions, Avulsions and Lacerations

Injury	Description	Signs and Symptoms	Treatment
Abrasions	A skin friction wound that involves one or more layers of the epidermis to be removed	Pain, redness and minor bleeding	Wound irrigation and debridement. Abrasions are kept moist to aid healing A non-adherent, sterile dressing is placed over the wound.
Avulsions	Avulsions are the traumatic tearing away and loss of the epidermis and dermis	Pain, bleeding and skin integrity alterations	Wound irrigation and debridement Approximation of wound edges is not possible Severe injuries may require skin grafting
Lacerations	The skin is torn or cut and separated without other tissue loss	Pain and bleeding	Irrigation and debridement Sutures may be necessary for deep lacerations and those over moving joints; wound closure strips can be used for superficial lacerations For 48 hours after closure a non-adherent dressing should be applied until epithelial bridging has taken place

Gunshot Wounds

Gunshot wounds can be purposeful, such as occurs with a crime, or accidental. Bullet wounds can come from high or low velocity bullets.

Signs and Symptoms

Gunshot injuries vary in terms of their character and intensity as based on the type of bullet, the type of the firearm and the distance from the firearm.

The bullet's yaw is the amount of distance that the bullet travels in an angular, rather than straight, path; the tumbling action of the bullet describes it turning, twisting and rotation of the bullet when it enters the body. Fragmentation is the splintering and breaking apart of pieces of the bullet when it enters the body. Yawing, tumbling and fragmentation increase the surface area of body tissue that the bullet contacts, which increases the damage's severity.

Bullet wounds are assessed in terms of their external and internal damages. The entry and exit wounds of a bullet can, in many circumstances, indicate what organs and other bodily structures, such as bones, can be affected. Entry wounds are usually oval or round and exit wounds typically appear like an irregular star. Entry wounds from close range are also characterized by a burn "tattoo".

Treatment

The treatment of gunshot wounds is driven by the extent of the damage and the priorities of care. For example, potentially fatal gunshot wounds require advanced life support measures, after which other wounds are managed and treated.

Paintball Gun Injuries

The vast majority of paintball injuries, which are blunt force injuries, include ocular damage and minor skin bruising and ecchymosis.

Signs and Symptoms

Superficial, soft tissue trauma presents with redness and bruising of the skin. Ocular injuries vary according to the intensity and location of the injury. Some of the most commonly occurring ocular injuries secondary to paint ball trauma include lens damage, hyphema formation, ocular neuropathy, choroidal rupture and angle recession.

Treatment

Common treatments for these injuries include cataract extraction and other interventions with ocular trauma. With, and without treatment, many of these preventable injuries can lead to blindness and the loss of an eye. Protective eye gear is highly recommended to prevent these injuries.

126

Nail Gun Injuries

Nail gun injuries are usually accidental and related to one's occupation. For example, construction workers frequently use nail guns. Most of these injuries affect the lower limbs but they can also lead to head, eye, dental, and other traumatic injuries.

Signs and Symptoms

The signs and symptoms of nail gun injuries vary according to the specific trauma that the nail has caused. For example, a penetrating nail gun injury in the skull will most likely be accompanied by neurological signs and symptoms of an intracranial bleed as well as external bleeding in the area. Similarly, a penetrating nail gun injury to the lower extremity will present with bleeding, pain, and possible skeletal trauma.

Treatment

Treatment varies according to the location, intensity of the injury. For example, penetrating head trauma is treated as a closed head injury, and skeletal injuries are treated as described above.

Pressure Ulcers

Pressure ulcers (also called pressure sores or bedsores) are injuries that occur due to excessive pressure on the skin. They can affect both the surface of the skin as well as the tissues that surround the area. Pressure ulcers are more common in areas that are bony, such as ankles, heel, hips or buttocks. Pressure ulcers form easily on people who are unable to move themselves easily, such as those who are wheelchair-bound, or those who are bedridden. The reason is that ulcers form when constant pressure is applied to one spot without relief.

Persons in a wheelchair most commonly develop pressure ulcers on their tailbone or buttocks, shoulder blades and spine. For those who are bedridden, the most common areas are heels, ankles and skin behind the knees, the rim of the ears, back or sides of the head, shoulder or shoulder blades, hip, lower back or tailbone.

Signs and Symptoms

There are four stages, based on severity, in which pressure ulcers fall. These stages are defined by The National Pressure Ulcer Advisory Panel, and are as follows:

1. Stage I: Skin is still intact. On people with lighter skin, it is reddish in color and does not blanch when pressure is applied to it. People with darker skin may not experience any change in the skin color of the affected area; furthermore, the affected skin does not blanch. The affected area of skin may appear purple or blue, or ashen. In comparison with the surrounding skin, the affected area may be particularly soft, firm, warmer, cooler, or more painful to the touch.

2. Stage II: The ulcer presents as an open wound. In other words, the entire epidermis (the exposed, outer layer of skin) and even part of the dermis (the underlying, unexposed layer of skin) is injured, damaged, or gone entirely. A pressure ulcer may appear pink or red and present as a shallow, basin-like wound or as fluid-filled blister (intact or ruptured).

3. Stage III: The ulcer presents as a deep wound, to the point that fat is exposed due to loss of skin. The ulcer appears deeper than the basin-like appearance described above and may be crater-like. Slough (yellowish dead tissue) may be visible at the bottom of the wound. There may be damage past the primary wound even below layers of seemingly healthy skin.

4. Stage IV: The ulcer shows major tissue loss; muscle, tendons, and even bone may be exposed. Slough or eschar (dark, crusty dead tissue) likely appears in the bottom of the wound. Damage often extends below layers of healthy skin past the primary wound.

Prevention of pressure sores requires repositioning, skin care, regular inspections and proper nutrition. Repositioning is essential and must occur frequently. For those who are wheelchair-bound or bedridden this can be difficult to do on their own, so it may require help. Those in a wheelchair need to move every fifteen minutes and the use of extra cushioning can help. For the bedridden, repositioning should occur every two hours and to assist they can use repositioning devices, special supportive mattresses and/or bed elevation, and protecting their bony areas is a must.

There are also a number of complications associated with pressure ulcers. Some examples are sepsis, cellulites, infections of the bone and /or joint, and cancer, such as a type of squamous cell carcinoma.

Treatment

With conservative care of the wound, stage I and II pressure sores will heal within several weeks to months. Pressure sores that are stage III and IV are harder to treat. If the patient also has a terminal illness, the treatment may focus more on pain relief as opposed to treating the sore itself.

When treating a pressure sore, there are different options, and sometimes a patient requires a combination of options. Specific treatments include pressure relief, which includes repositioning and support services; and removal of damaged tissue, which includes surgical debridement, mechanical debridement, autolytic debridement or enzymatic debridement. Other treatments include pain management, cleaning and dressing wounds, a healthy diet, antibiotics, muscle spasm relief, and surgical repair.

Puncture Wounds

A puncture wound is caused by an object or projectile, such as a nail, that penetrates the skin and underlying structures and tissues.

Signs and Symptoms

These wounds are typified with a small skin opening and very little bleeding. Despite the lack of signs and symptoms, however, they are highly susceptible to infection.

Treatment

Treatment includes stopping the blood, cleaning and applying a clean bandage for minor wounds; and surgical interventions may be necessary for more severe puncture wounds. Tetanus shots are necessary if the patient is not current.

De-gloving Injuries

De-gloving injuries are traumatic avulsion skin traumas. These injuries include the tearing away of the dermis and the epidermis.

Signs and Symptoms

De-gloving injuries are characterized by the pulling away of the skin's epidermis and dermis over a large area such as around the leg, foot or hand. These injuries are often accompanied by patient pain and anxiety.

Treatment

Treatment includes wound irrigation and debridement. These are typically not sutured, but covered with sterile dressing. Large areas may need skin grafting.

Psychosocial Emergencies

Abuse and Neglect

Abuse and neglect can be physical, psychological, and/or financial. Physical abuse can present as bruises, bone fractures, burns, etc. Sexual abuse includes any sexual contact with a minor or a person, even a spouse, who has not consented. Psychological abuse includes verbal bullying and threats of harm. Financial abuse can consist of withholding funds from another person.

Examples of neglect are the deprivation of adequate food (physical neglect), isolation and imprisonment in the home (psychological neglect), and a failure to provide another with sufficient funds to purchase things like shampoo even when there are ample funds to buy it (financial neglect).

All states have mandatory reporting laws. Nurses are mandated to report suspected child abuse or neglect, patient abuse or neglect, domestic violence and elder abuse and neglect. Mandated reporters are immune from civil and criminal liability due to reporting of any form of abuse, so long as the report is for a valid reason.

Anxiety

The North American Nursing Diagnosis Association (NANDA) defines anxiety as feelings of dread, discomfort, and apprehension. Anxiety leads to autonomic responses and the anticipation of danger.

Anxiety can be categorized as mild, moderate, severe and at panic level. Anxiety can also be further classified as death anxiety. This anxiety commonly affects those with terminal illnesses like cancer. Death anxiety is characterized by various degrees of dread and discomfort. The patient may express fears about the events surrounding death like incontinence and the loss of cognitive abilities, fears about pain at the time of death, uncertainty regarding encountering a higher power, and fears about the impact of their death on family members, among other things.

Signs and Symptoms

The signs and symptoms of anxiety include affective (increased helplessness, irritability, fright and worry), behavioral (insomnia and vigilance), sympathetic (anorexia, increased pulse, blood pressure and pulse), physiological (diaphoresis and trembling), parasympathetic (fatigue, urinary changes, weakness and faintness) and cognitive (poor problem solving skills and a lack of an adequate attention span).

Treatment

The nurse should assess the level of anxiety for both the patient and the significant other. As based on this assessment, some of the treatments can include empathy when the anxiety is rationale, encouraging the person to ventilate their feelings and perceptions, explaining all procedures, and using some techniques like cognitive/behavioral therapy, relaxation techniques, positive self-talk, massage and therapeutic touch.

Anxiety Disorders

Anxiety disorders are marked with characteristic physiological symptoms and responses. Some of the most commonly encountered anxiety disorders include panic disorder, obsessive-compulsive disorder, generalized anxiety disorder, social anxiety disorder, and phobias.

Anxiety disorders can completely consume the patient and make them unable to enjoy and/or participate in the activities of normal living. Although the cause of anxiety disorders is not fully understood, it appears that they, like so many other physical and emotional disorders, are the result of several factors. For example, anxiety disorders can occur as the result of a combination of stressful life events and personality traits like excessive worrying and ungrounded, irrational fears.

131

Signs and Symptoms

Anxiety can be classified as mild, moderate, severe and at panic level. Some of the presenting characteristics of mild anxiety include tension-diffusing behaviors like fidgeting and hair twisting, irritability, mild agitation, restlessness, attention-seeking behaviors, and mild, slight discomfort and uneasiness.

Some of the signs of moderate anxiety are shaking, impairments of memory, poor concentration, decreased attention span, voice tremors, increased respiratory rate, tachycardia, increased muscle tension, that may lead to headaches and backaches, and pacing and other forms of extreme tension, such as wringing of the hands.

The signs of severe anxiety are typically hyperventilation, tachycardia, hypertension, shortness of breath and other respiratory symptoms, rapid speech, feeling of impending doom and dread, confusion, and somatic complaints and signs of dizziness, nausea, vomiting, headache and sleeplessness.

The signs and symptoms associated with panic-level anxiety include pupil dilation, severe dizziness, tremors, chest pain, heart palpitations, immobility, feelings of absolute terror and fear, severe hyperactivity and possible physical exhaustion, an inability to speak and communicate with others, hallucinations, and delusions.

Treatment

Minor tranquilizers such as diazepam, clorazepate, and lorazepam are used to control, but not cure, overwhelming anxiety in the emergency department.

The emergency nurse will also initiate psychiatric mental health strategies such as:

- Establishing and maintaining a trusting relationship with the patient and significant others

- Effectively establishing and maintaining open, honest and nonjudgmental communication with the patient and significant others

- Encouraging the patient to verbalize their beliefs about stressors in their life

- Encouraging the patient to effectively cope with the stressors that are present in their life

- Identifying and assessing the patient's coping mechanisms

- Facilitating the development of more effective and appropriate coping mechanisms, as indicated

- Discussing, and teaching the patient, about ways that they can better resolve conflicts

- Providing the patient with information about available community resources for ongoing and follow up care

- Some of the many effective coping mechanisms that should be taught to the patient include things such as:

  o Positive self-talk

  o Stress management techniques

  o Assertiveness and learning how to say "no"

  o Problem solving strategies and techniques

  o Time management skills

  o Conflict resolution strategies

  o Anger management techniques

  o Community living skills

The goal of treatment in the emergency department is to stabilize the patient and discharge them to the home and available community resources. In order to accomplish this goal, the emergency nurse must use techniques of cognitive behavioral therapy, including offering assurance to the patient and maximizing the patient's strength, rather than focusing on the patient's weaknesses. All members of the emergency department should collaboratively find ways that will enable the patient to cope in a better manner.

Treatment after discharge is typically a combination of cognitive behavioral therapy, medications and community support or recovery programs under the direction of a psychiatrist, psychologist, social worker and/or counselors.

Panic and Panic Attacks

Panic, a symptom of extremely high anxiety, usually has an abrupt and sudden onset. Emergency care aims to stabilize the patient so that they can overcome this panic attack and return to the home and community without symptoms.

Signs and Symptoms

The patient experiencing high levels of fear and panic is usually in fear of losing control over themselves and their circumstances; they are overwhelmed with pronounced thoughts of doom and unrelenting fear. Signs and symptoms include shaking, chest pain, dyspnea, palpitations, and hyperventilation.

Treatment

Emergency nurses have to assess and care for patients having a panic attack in a reassuring and calm manner. All unnecessary and/or distressing stimulation must be eliminated and avoided. De-escalation of the situation is also important. Help the patient focus on their breathing and try stress reduction strategies like deep, cleansing breathing and soothing imagery. The nurse also tells the patient that they are in a safe place. Oftentimes, a friend or family member can sit with the patient in order to assist in calming them down.

Bereavement

Loss, often associated with grief, is multidimensional. Loss can be actual, perceived, or anticipated. It occurs when a person has a significant change that causes the loss of something of value, when the person anticipates a loss and when the person has a perceived the loss of something of value. Grieving is a normal response that includes physical, emotional, spiritual, social and intellectual responses. Sources of loss can include an intrapersonal loss of self and one's bodily image, and extra-personal losses like the loss of savings with the costs of medical care. All losses affect the patient.

Perceived losses are those losses that are not verifiable by others. This perception, although faulty, still affects the person. People have anticipatory grief before an actual or perceived loss occurs. For example, a son may undergo severe anticipatory grief soon after his mother has been diagnosed with cancer. Similarly, a woman may have anticipatory loss relating to her loss of sexuality after a mastectomy.

<u>Theories and Conceptual Frameworks Relating to Grief and Loss</u>

- *Kubler Ross's Stages of Grieving* - Similar to the other theories of loss, grieving and death, Kubler Ross's stages of grieving includes denial, anger, bargaining, depression, and acceptance. Bargaining is a unique phase of this theory. During the bargaining stage, the patient negotiates and bargains to avoid the loss. Spiritual support is often helpful during this stage.

- *Engel's Stages of Grieving* - According to Engel, the stages of grieving are shock and disbelief, developing awareness, restitution, resolving the loss, idealization and outcome. During shock and disbelief, the patient denies the loss and refuses to accept it. Later the patient consciously acknowledges the loss and may even express anger towards others, including family members and healthcare professionals. During the resolution stage, the patient contemplates the loss and may accept a dependent role in terms of their support network. Patients' family members may deify or idealize the lost loved one, or may experience guilt and/or ambivalence. During the outcome phase of Engel's model, the person adjusts to the loss as based on the characteristics of the loss.

- *Sander's Phases of Bereavement* - The phases of bereavement, according to Sander's theory, are shock, awareness of the loss, conservation and withdrawal, healing or the turning point, and renewal. These phases are quite similar to Engel's with some variations. For example, during the conservation and withdrawal phase, the person will withdraw from others and attempt to restore their physical and emotional wellbeing; during the healing stage, the person will move from emotional distress to the point where they are able to learn how to live without the loved one. During the renewal phase, the person is able to independently live without the loved one.

Signs and Symptoms

The defining characteristics of grief can include sleep disturbances, altered immune responses, anger, blame, withdrawal, pain, panic, distress, suffering and alterations with neuroendocrine functioning.

Treatment

Nurses can assist the patient with the grieving process by encouraging the person to ventilate their feelings, encouraging effective coping strategies, involving the family and significant others in the care of the patient, and, when needed, referring the patient and significant others to sources of psychosocial and spiritual support.

Bipolar Disorder

Bipolar disorder, also referred to as manic-depressive illness, is likely due to genetics, brain dysfunction, and some abnormal brain development

Signs and Symptoms

The signs and symptoms of bipolar disorder include periods of excitation and elevated mood, referred to as the manic phase of this disorder, and periods of sadness and depression during the depressive phase of this disorder.

Signs and symptoms of mania can include a happy mood, restlessness, insomnia and loss of sleep, extreme irritability, loss of focus and easy distraction, rapid speech, racing thoughts, poor impulse control and impulsive, and often risky, behaviors. The signs and symptoms of the depressive phase include the signs of depression, such as feelings of sadness, hopelessness and helplessness, loss of interest in activities, poor concentration, suicidal thoughts, difficulty making decisions, restlessness, irritability and changes in the patient's eating and sleeping patterns.

Treatment

Although there is no cure for bipolar disorder, it can be successfully managed with a combination of medications and psychotherapy. Mood stabilizers like lithium, anticonvulsants such as valproic acid (Depakote), lamotrigine (Lamictal), gabapentin (Neurontin), topiramate (Topamax), and oxcarbazepine (Trileptal) and antipsychotic medications are often used. Some of the antipsychotic medications include antidepressants, olanzapine (Zyprexa), aripiprazole (Abilify), quetiapine (Seroquel), risperidone (Risperdal) and ziprasidone (Geodon).

Some of the psychotherapy treatments include cognitive behavioral therapy, family therapy, and psycho-education. Other treatments include electroconvulsive treatments and medications to induce and maintain sleep.

Depression

Depression, of varying degrees, often affects the patient and those close to the patient when the person is affected with a serious, terminal illness like cancer. Depression leads to physical, emotional and cognitive changes. Depressive disorder is a growing, pervasive, chronic mental illness that affects millions in the West.

Signs and Symptoms

The signs and symptoms of depression include feelings of hopelessness, helplessness, sadness, dejection, despair, sleep loss, listlessness, headache, weight loss, anorexia, social withdrawal, lack of sexual desire, crying, poor levels of concentration, poor decision making and problem solving skills, diminished performance, personality changes, and a lack of self-worth and self-esteem.

Treatment

The care and treatment for a depressed patient is multifaceted. The patient needs social support and sometimes, spiritual support. They benefit from cognitive behavioral therapy, and often medications such as antidepressants, as well as non-pharmacological approaches such as stress reduction and relaxation techniques.

Homicidal/Violent Emergencies

Any time a disturbed or distressed patient presents in the ER, the nurse will assess their degree of risk in terms of harm to self and/or others and their signs and/or symptoms in respect to their mental health status. All emergency nurses must be vigilant and ready to react to dangerous and life-threatening patient behaviors. Homicidal and violent behaviors are most often associated with mentally ill patients, users of psychoactive substances and/or personality disorders.

Signs and Symptoms

Some of the potential warning signs of aggressive and violent behavior include:

- Clenched fists

- Adopting a fighting stance

- Swearing and cursing

- Veiled threats of harm

- Overt threats of harm

- Verbal abuse

- Slamming and throwing objects

- Aggressive outburst for no apparent reason

Treatment

Preventive actions are undertaken and all staff involved with an aggressive or violent person must avoid all escalating provocation. It is of vital importance to stay extremely calm and to avoid staring at or staring down the person. Neither restraint nor seclusion are preferred methods of treatment. They are a last resort. They should only be used when all preventive measures have failed, and then, the least restrictive method of restraint is used only when the restraint or seclusion is necessary to protect the patient and/or others from imminent danger; these should be removed when the patient is no longer dangerous.

There are two kinds of restraints -physical and chemical restraints. Physical restraints include things like vests, arm and leg restraints, shackles and any other device that restricts the patient's movement and mobility. A chemical restraint is a medication such as diazepam, midazolam and haloperidol, which is used to sedate the patient.

Psychosis

Psychosis is a serious mental disorder in which one can suffer from delusions and/or hallucinations. These mental problems can cause one to lose contact with reality.

Signs and Symptoms

Early signs and symptoms of psychosis include depression, difficulty concentrating, anxiety, changes in sleep (too much or too little,) unusual thoughts or beliefs that are ongoing, and suspiciousness. In later stages, signs and symptoms include hallucinations, delusions, depression, anxiety, suicidal thoughts or actions, difficulty functioning and disorganized speech, such as switching topics erratically.

Treatment

Treatment for psychosis usually involves medications, such as antipsychotics and tranquilizers, and psychotherapy, such as cognitive behavior therapy.

Situational Crises

A situational crisis is some type of major event in one's life that causes or poses a threat to them. It can threaten one's physical, emotional, or social integrity. The event can include job loss, which can leave someone feeling that their life has no meaning, worthlessness, fear and/or anxiety about being able to obtain other work, fear and/or anxiety about finances, etc. It can also result from divorce, a life event that can adversely impact on the patient's psychological, social and financial stability.

Suicide

Most often, a patient attempting suicide is depressed. This depression can be previously diagnosed or undiagnosed at the time of the suicide attempt.

Signs and Symptoms

Some of the most commonly occurring signs of suicide include:

- Lack of interest in the future
- An overwhelming sense of guilt and/or shame
- A significant drop in school or work performance
- Written or spoken notices of suicide intention
- Saying goodbye
- Dramatic changes in the personality or appearance
- Irrational, bizarre behaviour
- Giving away possessions

- Putting affairs in order

- Change in eating or sleeping patterns

- Self-harming actions, such as overdoses, which can be lethal

Like suicidal ideation among patients at the end of life, the same thoughts may affect family members and significant others. For example, an elderly woman may contemplate suicide after losing her husband.

Treatment

Constant observation and the use of restraints or seclusion may be necessary when the risk of suicide and self-harm are high. The safety of the suicidal person is the MOST important initial intervention for a suicidal patient. Antidepressants are the commonly medications for those at risk of suicide. Anti-psychotics and anti-anxiety medications depend on the patient's status.

Respiratory Emergencies

Aspiration

Aspiration is defined as drawing in gastric contents and/or food into the oropharynx, or choking. Critically ill patients, comatose patients, heavily sedated patients, those with gastroparesis and/or a swallowing disorder, tube-fed patients, those on mechanical ventilation and those who are vomiting are at risk for the aspiration of gastric contents. At times, the volume aspirated is large, thus placing the patient at risk for severe respiratory compromise and/or aspiration pneumonia.

Signs and Symptoms

The conscious person may cough or choke. An unconscious patient may also present with respiratory distress and the obvious signs of gastric contents when suctioned.

Treatment

Aspiration can be prevented by keeping the head of the bed elevated at a minimum of 30 degrees unless contraindicated, the sparing use of sedatives, the assessment of tube placement among tube-fed patients, continuous, rather than bolus, tube feedings and the assessment/treatment of swallowing disorders. Patients with aspiration are treated according to the underlying cause and the severity. Often, prophylactic antibiotics are administered to prevent aspiration pneumonia, which is a commonly occurring complication of aspiration.

Asthma

Asthma occurs when the airway narrows and swells. Severe asthma attacks can be life threatening, therefore, emergency treatment is necessary. Asthma can be acute or chronic.

Signs and Symptoms

The signs and symptoms of asthma include excessive mucus production, dyspnea, coughing, wheezing, shortness of breath, and chest tightness or pain.

Treatment

Asthma treatment medications depend on age, symptoms and triggers. Bronchodilators, such as albuterol, levalbuterol and pirbuterol, are used to open swollen airways. Others include ipratropium and oral and IV corticosteroids.

Chronic Obstructive Pulmonary Disease

Chronic obstructive pulmonary disease is a progressive respiratory disorder that impairs breathing and bodily oxygenation. Although most people equate COPD with emphysema, COPD also includes chronic bronchitis. Most people who have COPD have both chronic bronchitis and emphysema. The greatest risk factor is cigarette smoking; other risk factors include secondhand smoke and long-term exposures to irritants such as chemicals, air pollution and dust.

With emphysema, the airways and air sacs lose their elasticity, become thickened and inflamed and produce large amounts of mucus, which can block the airways. Eventually, the alveoli are destroyed, compromising gas exchange and oxygenation. With chronic bronchitis, the lining of the airways is always irritated and inflamed, the lining thickens and mucus production is increased, making breathing difficult.

Treatment

The goals of treatment include the relief of symptoms, the halting of progression, preventing complications and improving oxygenation. Smoking cessation, the avoidance of respiratory irritants, a good diet and pulmonary exercise are recommended. Other treatments include the use of bronchodilators, glucocorticosteroids, pulmonary exercises and rehabilitation, oxygen supplementation, and surgery, including a bullectomy to remove air spaces that interfere with breathing; a lung volume reduction that eases breathing and removes affected lung tissue, allowing remaining lung tissue to expand; and lung transplant.

Medications include short and long acting β2 agonists and anticholinergics such as salbutamol (Ventolin), terbutaline, ipratropium and tiotropium. Corticosteroids are also used to decrease any inflammation, and antibiotics like erythromycin can decrease the frequency of exacerbations. Supplemental oxygen is also recommended for many patients.

Pneumonitis

Pneumonitis is the inflammation of lung tissue. Chemotherapy drugs and radiation can cause pneumonitis and the combination of the two further increases the risk.

Signs and Symptoms

The most common is shortness of breath. Others include cough, shortness of breath, fatigue, anorexia and weight loss.

Treatment

Avoiding chemicals that the patient is hypersensitive to is an obvious treatment for pneumonitis. In more severe cases, treatment can include antibiotics for a bacterial infection, corticosteroids, such as prednisone, to reduce the inflammation, and oxygen therapy. If left untreated, it can develop into chronic pneumonitis.

Pneumonia

Pneumonia is an infection that inflames one or both lungs. Viruses, bacteria, fungi, and other organisms can cause pneumonia. While pneumonia may range from mild to life-threatening, it most strongly impacts infants and young children, the elderly, and patients with underlying health problems or weakened immunity.

Signs and Symptoms

The air sacs may fill with fluid or pus, resulting in cough with phlegm and difficulty breathing. These symptoms are generally accompanied by fever and chills. Others include muscular aches, fatigue, enlarged lymph nodes, a sore throat and chest pain. At times, bacterial pneumonia may have no symptoms.

Treatment

Includes antibiotics, fluids and oxygen supplementation, as indicated.

Inhalation Injuries

The most commonly occurring respiratory inhalation injuries occur from household cleaning agents; however, fire smoke, acts of terrorism and industrial gases such as chlorine and ammonia can also cause an inhalation injury.

Signs and Symptoms

These vary according to the agent and the volume/duration of the inhalation. They include respiratory distress and acute airway and lung obstruction, which can lead to death. Lung inflammation, bronchospasm, pulmonary edema, sloughing of tissue and scar formation can also occur in the respiratory passages and the lungs. Corrosive agents can lead to hemorrhage and permanent, irreversible scarring.

Treatment

The goal of treatment is to maintain adequate oxygenation. Analgesic medications, corticosteroids, oxygen, bronchodilators, humidification, and ventilators can help.

Respiratory Obstruction

An acute upper airway obstruction can occur from many causes including a foreign body, chemicals, throat cancer, allergic reactions such as anaphylaxis, respiratory infections such as pneumonia, epiglottitis, abscesses and croup.

Signs and Symptoms

Some of the signs and symptoms of a respiratory tract obstruction are apnea, coughing, agitation, cyanosis, unconsciousness, panic, air hunger and unusual respiratory noises such as crowing, whistling and wheezing.

Treatment

Emergency measures such as the Heimlich are performed for complete airway obstruction. Other treatments include oxygen administration, foreign body removal, an endotracheal or nasotracheal tube and mechanical ventilation, as indicated.

Pleural Effusion

Pleural effusion is a collection of fluid in the pleural space around the lung caused by excessive fluid production or a decrease in fluid absorption. A pleural effusion can occur in almost any type of cancer, but the most common causes of a malignant pleural effusion are lung and breast cancer. Pleural effusion can be the first sign of cancer, a reoccurrence of cancer or advanced stages of cancer.

Signs and Symptoms

Possible signs and symptoms include dyspnea, cough, chest pain and fever.

Treatment

The treatment of pleural effusion requires treating an underlying condition. For example, if bacterial pneumonia is present, antibiotics can help. Drainage is often required if the pleural effusion is extensive, infected or inflamed. Other treatment methods include chest tubes to drainage and thoracentesis.

Pneumothorax and Hemothorax

A pneumothorax, or collapsed lung, occurs when there is leakage of air or fluid into the area between the chest wall and the lungs. This abnormal collection of air or fluid leads to pressure on the lung, which can cause it to collapse. A hemothorax has the same signs and symptoms as a pneumothorax, but a hemothorax occurs as the result of blood leaking into the area that occurs, for example, with trauma.

Signs and Symptoms

These include chest pain and shortness of breath.

Treatment

Relieving the pressure on the lung is the ultimate goal of treatment for a pneumothorax. In some cases, such as with a partially collapsed lung, the physician may choose to administer supplemental oxygen and monitor the patient to see if the air is reabsorbed and the lung reinflates. Serious cases may require aspiration, chest tube placement to remove the air, and the surgical repair of the leaking area.

Pulmonary Edema

Pulmonary edema occurs when the alveoli of the lung(s) fill with fluid, thus preventing exchanges of carbon dioxide and oxygen. Pulmonary edema can be caused by many different factors including heart failure, which is referred to as cardiogenic pulmonary edema, and other causes that are not cardiogenic.

Signs and Symptoms

The signs and symptoms of pulmonary edema include dyspnea, shortness of breath, abnormal breath sounds, fatigue, cyanosis, tachypnea and hypoxia.

Treatment

The treatment of pulmonary edema is primarily based on the underlying cause and its severity. Some treatments include diuretics, oxygen supplementation, suctioning, mechanical ventilation and antibiotics when it is caused by infection.

Pulmonary Embolus

Pulmonary emboli most often occur as the result of deep vein thrombosis in the legs or thigh. Other less likely causes include a fat embolus post-skeletal bone fracture, air bubbles and tumors.

Signs and Symptoms

Some of the signs and symptoms include shortness of breath, dyspnea, chest pain, coughing, tachypnea, tachycardia, hypoxia, cyanosis, anxiety and panic.

Treatment

This condition is an emergency that requires rapid treatment. Thrombolytic therapy with streptokinase or a tissue plasminogen activator, anticoagulation therapy to prevent new clot formation and oxygen supplementation can help.

Acute Respiratory Distress Syndrome (ARDS)

ARDS is caused by pneumonia, sepsis, trauma, chemical inhalation and aspiration.

Signs and Symptoms

The signs and symptoms include dyspnea, shortness of breath, abnormal breath sounds, fatigue, cyanosis, tachypnea, hypotension, hypoxia, and hypotension. It can lead to multisystem failure and compromise.

Treatment

Patients are hospitalized in a special care area for intubation, mechanical ventilation, oxygen supplementation, and the treatment of any underlying causes.

Tension Pneumothorax

A tension pneumothorax usually occurs as the result of trauma, such as a laceration of the lung, which leads to a build-up of air in the pleural space.

Signs and Symptoms

These include a shift of the trachea and the mediastinum to the opposite side of the tension pneumothorax, hyperextension of the chest, hypoxia, tachycardia, tachypnea, hypotension and circulatory collapse.

Treatment

Emergency treatment of a tension pneumothorax includes rapid chest decompression with a needle thoracotomy and chest tube placement.

Environmental Emergencies

Burns

Burns are classified according to their depth and level of involvement.

Signs and Symptoms

1. A first-degree burn is superficial, and typically heals in a couple of days without scarring. However, they are painful.

2. A second-degree burn is a partial thickness injury consisting of the epidermis and the upper dermis. These burns are more painful than a third-degree burn, which is more severe. There is blistering and, depending on depth (superficial or deep partial injury), it may need grafting. These appear as red or pale red.

3. A third-degree burn injury destroys all layers of the skin and affects some underlying tissue (bone, muscle and nerves). There is no blistering; these burns require grafting and excision. The result of a full thickness injury is that the center is surrounded by layers: A coagulation area, then a stasis area, then an area of erythema, all of which are surrounded by normal tissue.

The Lund and Browder chart is the most accurate method of determining the extent of burns in a pediatric patient. It is based on age and the estimated percentage of total body surface area (TBSA) affected. In pediatrics, a minor burn is a first- or second-degree burn that covers 10% or less of the TBSA. Moderate burns are second-degree burns that cover 10-20% of the TBSA or third-degree burns that cover 2-5% and do not affect the face, hands, feet, or genitals.

Major burns include:

- Any burns on the face or head, feet, hands, or genitals

- Electrical burns

- Any second-degree burn covering 20% or more of the TBSA

- Any third degree burn covering 5-10% of the TBSA

- Any minor-moderate burn with additional trauma, fractures or complications

The Rule of Nines for Adult Burns

The rule of nines aids in a quick estimation of burn size until a more thorough assessment is feasible. The anterior and posterior portion of each leg is 9% and all other areas are multiples of 9%. For example, the anterior and posterior of each arm is 4.5%. The anterior and posterior chest is 18% and the anterior and posterior of the face/skull is 4.5%.

System-Wide Effects of Major Burns

- Hyperventilation and increased oxygen demand

- Too much fluid in the fluid resuscitation phase along with burn shock changes can cause pulmonary edema. If the patient has an inhalation burn injury, there may be a need to limit hydration to prevent this serious complication.

- The initial respiratory alkalosis from the hyperventilation may quickly change to respiratory acidosis associated with pulmonary insufficiency.

- Fluid shift causes lesser circulating blood volume, resulting in lower cardiac output and tachycardia

- A decreased stroke volume occurs and the increased blood viscosity and vasoconstriction of the arterioles causes a high peripheral resistance.

- Initial hyperkalemia is a result of cell death, followed by hypokalemia as fluid shifts deplete potassium that is not replaced in the vascular compartment. The outcome is inadequate tissue perfusion, which may lead to acidosis, renal failure, and irreversible "burn shock".

- Hyponatremia occurs between the 3rd and 10th day from fluid shifts.

- Catecholamine is released in response to burn injury and may be the major reason for the hyper-metabolic response to a burn injury. Glucose is the needed fuel for hyper-metabolism and stores in the liver and muscle are exhausted usually within the first few days; then, the liver must increase its gluconeogenesis. Insulin levels decrease early in the burn response and the patient will show hyperglycemia, probably due to the gluconeogenesis.

- Proteins from the muscles and viscera are mobilized to meet the need.

- Adequate fluid intake (electrolytes and intravenous solutions) will result in the patient gaining weight in the first few days. Three to four days later, the mobilization of the fluids (and excretion via the kidneys) and catabolic responses will cause this weight to fall off.

- 3,000-5,000 calories are needed to reverse negative nitrogen balance and promote a positive nitrogen balance necessary for healing. (A high protein, high calorie diet is necessary for a 10-20% burn; enteral feedings for supplementation are needed for a 20-30% burn; TBSA burns of 30-40% require total parenteral nutrition with lipids, called a "3-in-1" TPN solution).

- Metabolic need increases proportionally with TBSA. A burn of 40-50% would mean the metabolic rate is essentially double the normal rate.

- Red blood cells die from thermal injury and coagulate around areas of the burn. The total mass of RBCs in the vascular system is diminished from death, thrombosis formation, and sludging. As fluid shifts out of the vascular compartment, the hematocrit rises and blood flow is impaired in micro-circulation. Capillary stasis may cause further ischemia and even necrosis.

- Compensatory mechanisms for plasma volume losses include vasoconstriction, fluid shift out of undamaged extracellular spaces, and the sensation of thirst.

- The epidermis is a protective water vapor barrier and if it is nonfunctional, surface fluid loss becomes a problem causing fluid deficits.

- The fluid deficit is based on the amount of epidermis lost and the burn depth.

- Capillary permeability increases, allowing both fluid and albumin to leak into the interstitial spaces and out of the vascular system. This happens within the first 24-36 hours with a peak usually at the twelfth hour post-burn. The patient can go into a hypovolemic shock because of this fluid shifting.

- Protein rich fluids also weep out of second-degree burns and from the surface of full-thickness burns.

- About the 48th hour post-burn, the capillary permeability begins to change back. About 72 hours post-burn, the fluid shifts from the interstitial tissue to the intravascular system. At that time, the patients with good cardiac and renal function will show fluid diuresis. In patients with compromised renal or cardiac function, the fluid can overload, causing pulmonary edema.

- If "fluid resuscitation" post-burn is delayed or inadequate, renal blood flow decreases, which can lead to high output failure or oliguric renal failure with a decreased creatinine clearance.

- Glomerular filtration may be decreased in extensive burn responses.

- Deep muscle damage (due to an electrical burn) causes the hemoglobin and myoglobin to be released into the urine and may result in tubular necrosis unless increased fluids are given.

- Thrombocytopenia, impaired platelet function, decreased fibrinogen levels, diminished fibrinolysis, and inhibition of plasma clotting factors are characteristic of responses to major burn injuries.

- Destruction of red blood cells, a decreased life span of the remaining blood cells, and blood loss (covert or overt) lead to post-burn anemia.

- Decreased peristalsis can lead to nausea, vomiting, gastric distention, and paralytic ileus.

- The burn patient has an extremely high risk for gastric ulcers and duodenal ulcers from ischemic changes in the gastric mucosa. Bleeding via occult changes is common and hemorrhage is a major complication.

- Some major immunoglobulins diminish in response to burn injury.

- Decreases in cellular immunity are demonstrated by lymphocytopenia, impaired resistance to viruses, fungi, and gram-negative organisms.

- The destruction of the skin barrier favors bacterial growth while the formation of vascular granulation tissue resists bacteria. The inflammatory response results in decreased transport of white blood cells, oxygen, and antibiotics to the burn area but hypoxia, followed by acidosis and thrombosis of the vessels, cause an impaired resistance to bacterial invasion.

- Wound colonization by bacteria on the surface may progress to invasion of the adjacent non-burned and viable tissues. Usually, the surface of the wound is fully colonized in 3-5 days. Only a burn wound biopsy, a quantitative culture that demonstrates a bacterial count of 105 per gram of tissue indicates burn wound sepsis.

Treatment

The goals of fluid resuscitation are a urinary output of 30-50 ml/hour, a pulse rate less than 120 beats per minute, CVP readings, pulmonary artery end diastolic pressure in the low to normal range, and a stable mental state and level of consciousness.

The Parkland Formula is used to calculate fluid requirements among burn patients.

1. For the first 24 hours post burn, the fluid needs are calculated as follows:

2. 2-4 ml Lactated Ringer's solution X body weight (in Kg) X percent burn

3. Fluid is given as 50% in the first eight hours followed by 50% over the next 16 hours. An adult (75Kg) with a 50% TBSA example would look like this:

4. 4ml X 75 kg X 50 = 15,000 ml over the first 24 hours

5. 50% over the first eight hours = 7,500 mls, or (937.5) 938 mls per hour

6. 50% over the next 16 hours = (468.75) 469 mls per hour

7. Minor burns are treated with the application of silvadene ointment, cool compresses and hydrocortisone cream for pain, as well as NSAIDs.

8. Partial-thickness burns are cleaned and covered with a sterile dressing. Full-thickness burns usually require surgical interventions such as debridement and skin grafting. Major burns can cause infection and shock.

Insect Stings

Insect stings involve injected poisons that produce local and systemic reactions.

Signs and Symptoms

Local signs and symptoms include pain, erythema, edema, and itching; systemic reactions can be severe to life-threatening if the person has an anaphylactic reaction, which is characterized by unconsciousness, laryngeal edema, and cardiovascular collapse. Epinephrine and a bronchodilator are the drugs of choice for anaphylaxis.

Treatment

Remove the stinger by pulling it from the skin without squeezing, because this may cause additional venom to inject. Ice packs to the area and elevation of the extremity help if there is a large edematous local reaction. Oral antihistamines should be given and the site cleansed with soap and water. A tetanus vaccination may be appropriate.

Wound care starts after the patient has been assessed and treated for possible shock and poisoning. Shaving the surrounding area allows for better visualization of the area, and for the effective adhesion of dressings to the skin. The wound should be gently irrigated with copious amounts of isotonic sterile saline or sterile water to remove debris. A catheter-tip syringe (an irrigation/bulb syringe) may be used. If the wound is grossly contaminated, the physician may need to anesthetize the wound before proceeding. Then, a surgical scrub with antiseptic is followed by copious amounts of sterile solution. Removal of devascularized tissue or tissue impeding healing will promote healthy re-growth of granulation tissue. A wound requiring primary closure will need sutures, staples, or skin adhesives/tape.

Wound dressing consist of three layers - a non-adherent layer against the surface of the wound, an absorbent layer, and a cover layer that keeps the dressing in place; this may be a gauze wrap or pad. Infection potential of an open wound is always a concern. Antibiotic ointment helps minor wounds while IV antibiotics may be needed for major wounds. Elevation of the affected extremity for the first 48 hours will assist the healing process by reducing the amount of edema; the patient should be instructed to sleep with the head of the bed elevated if facial wounds are present.

Poisonous Animal Bites

Bites from rattlesnakes, copperheads and coral snakes are most common in the US.

Signs and Symptoms

In addition to a puncture wound, the patient may show the signs of severe cardiac and respiratory compromise.

Treatment

Assess the ABCs and be prepared for resuscitation. Watch for signs of local reactions such as burning, itching, swelling at the site, blisters and extremity edema and discoloration; assess for systemic reactions including nausea, diaphoresis, light-headedness, euphoria followed by drowsiness, difficulty swallowing, dyspnea, and muscle paralysis. The affected area should be kept below the level of the heart. Other treatments include the use of Sawyer pump suctioning, and the administration of antivenom, as listed below.

Snake Antivenoms

Antivenom	Species	Country
Polyvalent snake antivenom	South American Rattlesnake *Crotalus durissus* and fer-de-lance *Bothrops asper*	Mexico
Polyvalent snake antivenom	Saw-scaled Viper *Echis carinatus*, Russell's Viper *Daboia russelli*, Spectacled Cobra *Naja naja*, Common Krait *Bungarus caeruleus*	India
Polyvalent crotalid antivenin (CroFab Crotalidae Polyvalent Immune Fab (Ovine))	North American pit vipers (rattlesnakes, copperheads, and cottonmouths)	North America
Soro antibotropicocrotalico	Pit vipers and rattlesnakes	Brazil, USA
Antielapidico	Coral snakes	Brazil, USA
SAIMR polyvalent antivenom	Mambas, Cobras, Rinkhalses, Puff Adders	South Africa
Panamerican serum	Coral snakes	Costa Rica
Anticoral	Coral snakes	Costa Rica
Anti-mipartitus antivenom	Coral snakes	Costa Rica
Anticoral monovalent	Coral snakes	Costa Rica
Coralmyn	Coral snakes	Mexico
Anti-micruricoscorales	Coral snakes	Colombia

Other Antivenoms

Antivenom	Species	Country
Soro antiloxoscelico	Recluse spider	Brazil
Aracmyn	Recluses and Black Widows	Mexico/USA
Black widow antivenom	Black widow spider	United States
Anti Latrodectus antivenom	Black Widow spider	Argentina
zoro antilonomico	Giant Silkworm Moth (Caterpillar)	Brazil
Alacramyn	Bark scorpions,	Mexico
Suero Antialacran	*Centruroides limpidus, C. noxius, C. suffusus*	Mexico
Soro antiscorpionico	*Tityus spp.*	Brazil
SAIMR scorpion antivenin	*Parabuthus spp.*	South Africa

Food Poisoning

Food poisoning, also referred to as food-borne illness, is an illness that results from eating contaminated food. The most common type of contamination is infectious organisms, including bacteria, viruses, parasites and/or their toxins. Food contamination can occur during any part of processing or production. Contamination can also occur in the home, if foods are not properly handled and cooked.

Signs and Symptoms

Food poisoning signs and symptoms can appear within hours of eating or up to days or weeks after. The common symptoms include nausea, vomiting, diarrhea, abdominal pain and cramps, and a fever. Other symptoms that are far more serious include vomiting frequently with an inability to keep liquids down, vomiting blood, severe diarrhea for 3 days or more, blood present in bowel movements, a temperature of 101.5F or higher, signs of dehydration, trouble speaking, trouble swallowing, double vision, and muscle weakness.

Treatment

Depending on the severity, treatment can vary. In some cases, it goes away in a few days or a week or more. Treatment can include fluid replacement and antibiotics for certain types of bacterial food poisoning, accompanied by severe symptoms. Intravenous antibiotics must be given as soon as possible for those with food poisoning by listeria. Antibiotics are often used in women who are pregnant and suffer from food poisoning in order to prevent the infection from harming the fetus.

Organophosphates and Insecticides

Organophosphate poisoning causes the inhibition of acetylcholinesterase in the body and acetylcholine to accumulate. Organophosphate poisoning is generally the consequence of insecticide exposure; however, it can also occur with bioterrorism nerve agents. Suicides and suicidal attempts are often done with organophosphates and other insecticides.

Signs and Symptoms

These include polyuria, constricted pupils, increased salivation, tearing, diarrhea, abdominal cramps, anorexia, nausea, vomiting, bradycardia, dyspnea, coma, convulsions, and cyanosis.

SLUDGEM (salivation, lacrimation, urination, defecation, gastrointestinal motility, emesis, miosis) and MUDDLES (miosis, urination, diarrhea, diaphoresis, lacrimation, excitation, and salivation) are two mnemonics that make the signs and symptoms relatively easy to remember.

Treatment

Antidotes like atropine can be used in this life-threatening situation.

Giardia

Giardia infection, known as giardiasis, is caused by a parasite that is most commonly found in areas with poor sanitation and unsafe water. This infection is waterborne, and can be found anywhere from backcountry streams or lakes to swimming pools and spas. It is also transmitted through food and person-to-person contact.

Signs and Symptoms

In some cases, people are just carriers, but they can infect others that may come in contact with their stool. The symptoms include watery, foul smelling diarrhea, fatigue, malaise, abdominal cramps and bloating, nausea, weight loss, and belching gas with a bad taste. These symptoms usually last for two to four weeks.

Treatment

Mild cases usually go away on their own, whereas severe cases are treated with antibiotic medications, such as metronidazole, tinidazole and nitazoxanide.

Ringworm

Ringworm, also referred to as tinea, is a fungal skin infection. It often presents as several patches on the skin at one time.

Signs and Symptoms

Signs and symptoms include itchy, raised, scaly patches with defined edges that can blister and ooze. These patches often appear as a reddened ring surrounded by normal colored skin tissue. If it affects the nails they will be thick discolored and often crumble; if it affects the hair, it causes bald patches.

Treatment

Severe cases and those that last a long time or that affect the hair are treated with medication, such as ketoconazole. Antibiotics may be prescribed if a skin infection occurs from excessive scratching.

Tapeworms

Tapeworm infestation occurs when food or water is contaminated with tapeworm eggs or larvae. Invasive infection occurs when the tapeworm eggs migrate outside of the intestines and form larval cysts in bodily tissue or organs.

In an intestinal infection, the affected person (the host) has ingested tapeworm larvae which then developed into adult tapeworms in the host's intestines. An adult tapeworm has a head (which connects to the intestinal wall), a neck, and a series of segments called proglottids, which produce eggs. Adult tapeworms may live in the host's intestines for up to twenty years. Intestinal infections are usually mild, but invasive larva infections are serious.

Signs and Symptoms

Intestinal tapeworms usually cause no signs and symptoms, but if they do, they include nausea, weakness, diarrhea, a loss of appetite, weight loss, abdominal pain, and malnutrition from an inability to absorb adequate nutrients from food. Invasive infections, when larvae migrate from the intestines and form cysts in other tissues, eventually lead to organ and tissue damage. Symptoms include fever, allergic reactions, bacterial infections, cystic masses or lumps, and seizures.

Treatment

Many ringworms will exit the body on their own, whereas others need treatment. Medications, such as praziquantel, albendazole, and nitazoxanide, are toxic to ringworms. Reinfection may occur so follow up stool samples are taken and education on hand washing should be given. For invasive infections, depending on the location and effects of the infection, anthelmintic drugs such as albendazole may be used to shrink the cyst. If the tapeworm is dying, anti-inflammatory therapy and corticosteroids, such as prednisone or dexamethasone, may be indicated. Seizures from the disease can be treated with anticonvulsant medications.

Pinworms

Pinworms are the most common type of intestinal worm. They are thin, white, and measure 5-13mm in length. They are most common among school-age children.

Signs and Symptoms

Some people have no symptoms, but those who do may experience itching of the anus or vaginal area, insomnia or restlessness, pain and nausea.

Treatment

Treatments include anti-parasite medication such as mebendazole or albendazole. Oftentimes the medication is given to all the members of the household.

Lice

Lice are tiny, parasitic insects that feed on blood. Lice can be found on the head, the body, and the pubic area, which are referred to commonly as "crabs".

Signs and Symptoms

Signs and symptoms include itching and small, red bumps on the scalp, neck and shoulders. Adult lice are the size of a sesame seed and the nits resemble dandruff.

Treatment

Treatment for head lice includes a special over-the-counter shampoo, Malathion, or benzyl alcohol lotion or lindane.

Maggot Infestation (Myiasis)

Myiasis is classified according to the area affected. These classifications include dermal, sub-dermal, cutaneous, nasopharyngeal, ocular, auricular, gastrointestinal and urogenital myiasis.

Signs and Symptoms

- *Aural Myiasis* - The patient may report buzzing in their ear. Ear discharge, if present, may be foul smelling. The larvae can enter the brain when the middle and inner ear are affected.

- *Cutaneous Myiasis* - Painful boils that can last for an extensive period.

- *Ophthalmomyiasis* - Eye irritation, pain and edema

- *Nasal Myiasis* - Nasal congestion and obstruction, fever, and facial edema

Treatment

The surgical removal of the larva requires a local anesthetic, such as lidocaine, and forceps. After removal, the site is dressed and antibiotics are often given to prevent a secondary infection. Another treatment, although not preferred, occludes and suffocates the larva. Cutaneous myiasis is treated with a thick coat of petroleum jelly to rob the larva of their oxygen supply, which then moves them to the surface for relatively simple removal. All types of myiasis can be treated with oral ivermectin (200 mcg/kg) ivermectin or topical ivermectin (1% solution).

Scabies

An itchy skin condition caused by *Sarcoptes scabiei*, a tiny burrowing mite, is known as scabies. This condition is contagious and can it can spread quickly.

Signs and Symptoms

These include itchiness, often worse at night, and thin, irregular burrow tracks made up of tiny blisters or bumps on the skin. In adults, it is mostly found between fingers, in armpits, on the inner elbow, soles of the feet, around breasts, around the male genital area, along the insides of wrists, and around the waist. In children, it is commonly seen on the scalp, face, neck, palms of the hands and soles of the feet.

Treatment

Treatment includes medications, such as permethrin 5%, lindane, and crotamiton. For those that don't respond to lotions and creams, ivermectin is prescribed orally.

Contact Dermatitis

Contact dermatitis is a type of skin inflammation that occurs as the result of skin contacted a substance that causes irritation or an allergic reaction. These substances can include plants, such as poison ivy or poison oak, chemicals, and other substances.

Signs and Symptoms

These include a red rash or bumps, itchiness, skin that is dry and cracked, red patches that may look like a burn, blisters, which in severe cases drain fluid and crust, a skin rash to the exposed and affected area, pain and tenderness.

Treatment

Treatment includes avoiding the irritant or allergen, corticosteroid creams, wet compresses and oral medications such as corticosteroids or antihistamines.

Plant Ingestion

Many plants and plant parts can be poisonous to humans and other animals.

Signs and Symptoms

The signs and symptoms vary according to the ingested plant or plant part.

- *Hemlock* - Hemlock poisoning becomes symptomatic in fifteen minutes. Dry mouth, respiratory compromise, tachycardia, tremors, diaphoresis, mydriasis, seizures, and muscle paresis. Bradycardia and rhabdomyolysis may also occur.

- *Foxglove and Oleander* - Gastroenteritis, hyperkalemia, confusion, and arrhythmias can occur. Serum digoxin levels can confirm the diagnosis.

- *Castor Beans and Jequirity Beans* - Symptoms include delayed gastroenteritis, hemorrhage, delirium, seizures, coma, and death.

- *Aconitine* - Symptoms include bradycardia, paresthesia, dysrhythmias, and weakness

- *Aloe* - Symptoms include gastroenteritis, nephritis, skin irritation

- *Birthworts and Pipevines* - Tubulointerstitial nephropathy can occur

- *Azalea* - Cholinergic symptoms

- *Elephant Ears* - The leaves lead to oral mucosal damage due to calcium oxalate crystals

Treatment

- *Hemlock* - Aggressive supportive symptomatic treatments are necessary. The ABCs are priority. Other treatments include gastric lavage, activated charcoal, seizure precautions, benzodiazepine for seizures, aggressive fluid replacement, intubation and mechanical ventilation, as indicated.

- *Foxglove* - Activated charcoal, ventilator support, fluid replacement and gastric lavage

- *Castor Beans and Jequirity Beans* - Whole bowel irrigation is necessary to remove the beans.

- *Oleander* - Ventilator support, fluid replacement, activated charcoal and gastric lavage are treatment options

- *Aconitine* - Treatment includes supportive care and atropine

- *Aloe* - Supportive care and irrigation are treatment options

- *Birthworts and Pipevines* - Supportive care

- *Azalea* - Supportive care and atropine

- *Elephant Ears* - Airway maintenance and other supportive care

Radiation/Hazardous Material Exposure

Some of the external factors that affect health include variables like climate, air and water quality, environment toxins and substances like asbestos, radiation, and sulfur dioxide found in acid rain. Ionizing radiation is considered an environmental risk factor associated with cancer. Ionizing radiation comes from rays that enter the earth's atmosphere from outer space, radioactive fallout, radon gas, x-rays, therapeutic radiation for cancer, and other sources.

Radiation safety is based on the three principles of time, distance and shielding. You must minimize the time, or duration, of the exposure; you must also create and maximize the distance between the person and the source of the radiation; shielding, with lead aprons and gloves, is needed for protection.

Radon gas, which can't be seen, smelled or tasted, is found in many homes and buildings, especially in the South and on the West Coast.

Many studies have shown that exposure to asbestos, benzene, benzidine, cadmium, nickel, and vinyl chloride also may cause cancer. The Environmental Protection Agency (EPA) and the International Agency for Research on Cancer have declared asbestos a human carcinogen. Exposure can result in numerous types of cancer, but the two most common include mesothelioma and lung cancer. Studies have demonstrated that asbestos exposure is a risk factor for malignant mesothelioma, while other studies indicate a risk for lung cancer is related to the duration of exposure and cumulative dose. The carcinogeny of asbestos has resulted in its prohibition and/or regulation in most countries. However, humans are still threatened by direct or potential asbestos exposure.

Hypothermia

Hypothermia is defined as a core body temperature of less than 95 degrees. The greatest risk factor is prolonged exposure to cold, particularly in bodies of water. Heat production is less than heat losses. The elderly are at particular risk. Other risk factors include thyroid disease, trauma and diabetes.

Signs and Symptoms

The signs and symptoms include confusion, slurred speech, numbness, shivering, drowsiness, lethargy, shallow respirations and a loss of consciousness.

Treatment

This life-threatening condition is treated with the provision of warmth and other supportive measures. All wet clothing is removed, dry clothing and blankets are provided, warm fluids are provided, the trunk is warmed prior to the extremities and warm packs and a hyperthermia blanket may be applied.

Hyperthermia

Hyperthermia is an elevated bodily temperature above 99.5 degrees that is often described as "heat stroke". Prolonged exposure to heat, particularly humid heat, is the primary cause of hyperthermia. Other risk factors include some medications like selective serotonin reuptake inhibitors and monoamine oxidase inhibitors psychotropic drugs, prolonged, intensive exercise and activity, damage to the hypothalamus and central nervous system damage.

Signs and Symptoms

Some of the signs and symptoms of hyperthermia are vasodilation, hot, dry skin, dehydration, nausea, vomiting, hypotension, confusion, dizziness, tachycardia, tachypnea, seizures, coma and death when left untreated.

Treatment

Whenever possible, the underlying cause such be diagnosed and treated. Other treatments include hydration, the provision of coolness with wet packs or a hypothermia blanket, gastric lavage and cool, iced saline.

Rabies

Rabies is a deadly virus that infected animals spread to people through the animal's saliva. Rabid animals in the U.S. include bats, coyotes, foxes, raccoons and skunks.

Signs and Symptoms

Signs and symptoms of rabies can be similar to the flu, and they include fever, headache, nausea, vomiting, agitation, anxiety, confusion, hyperactivity, difficulty swallowing, excessive salivation, hydrophobia or fear of water related to the difficulty swallowing, insomnia, hallucinations, and partial paralysis.

Treatment

Rabies is highly fatal. Rabies immune globulin is administered and supportive care is provided.

Toxicological Emergencies

Sulfuric Acid Poisoning

Sulfuric acid is a very strong corrosive chemical that burns skin and mucous membrane tissue. Sulfuric acid is found in batteries, detergent, toilet bowel cleaners and some fertilizers.

Signs and Symptoms

The signs and symptoms associated with sulfuric acid ingestion are respiratory compromise, burns in the mouth and throat, convulsions, fever, pain, vomiting, sometimes with blood, and visual changes. Inhalation injuries present cyanosis, coughing, hypotension, tachycardia, shortness of breath, dyspnea and coughing up blood. Cutaneous contact is characterized by pain, skin redness and signs of a burn.

Treatment

Flushing the skin with copious amounts of water is helpful. Ingested sulfuric acid poisoning is treated with respiratory support, intravenous fluids, and surgical repair of damaged tissue. The patient remains NPO (no food or fluids allowed) and vomiting is *not* induced. Inhalation injuries are treated symptomatically.

Hydrochloric Acid Poisoning

Hydrochloric acid is a clear, corrosive substance that, like sulfuric acid, causes serious and often life-threatening tissue damage when ingested, inhaled or contacted. Hydrochloric acid is found in some fertilizers and pool chemicals.

Signs and Symptoms

Swallowing hydrochloric acid can lead to respiratory compromise, severe chest pain, fever, abdominal pain, excessive salivation, hypotension and vomiting of blood.

The signs and symptoms of inhalation include cyanosis, hypotension, tachycardia, chest tightness and pain, coughing up blood, shortness of breath, dyspnea and often severe respiratory compromise. Contact with the skin or mucus membranes causes pain, blisters and burns.

Treatment

Treatment for hydrochloric and sulfuric acid is identical.

Carbon Monoxide Poisoning

Carbon monoxide poisoning occurs when a patient is exposed to excessive carbon monoxide, diminishing their ability to absorb oxygen. This can lead to tissue damage and death. Carbon monoxide is odorless and colorless. The greatest risk factors for carbon monoxide poisoning are from buildings including private homes, and automobiles running in an enclosed area, such as a garage.

Signs and Symptoms

The signs and symptoms of carbon monoxide poisoning include nausea, vomiting, dizziness, weakness, a dull headache, shortness of breath, confusion, blurred vision, and loss of consciousness. People who are sleeping or intoxicated are especially in danger, as the fumes can be fatal prior to anyone realizing that a problem is present.

Treatment

Treatment includes administering pure oxygen through a facemask, or a ventilator, and in some cases, hyperbaric oxygen therapy may be necessary.

Cyanide Poisoning

Cyanide poisoning is rare; however, it makes the cells of the body unable to use oxygen, which can prove to be deadly.

Signs and Symptoms

Signs and symptoms of cyanide poisoning include weakness, confusion, bizarre behavior, excessive sleepiness, coma, shortness of breath, headache, dizziness, pink or cherry-red skin, very fast or slow heartbeat, breath smelling like almonds, and seizures. An acute ingestion has a rapid onset, which affects the heart immediately, causing sudden collapse. It can also affect the brain causing a seizure or coma. Chronic incidents have a gradual onset.

Treatment

Treatment for cyanide poisoning includes stomach pumping, hydroxocobalamin, and hyperbaric oxygen therapy. Cyanide poisoning is an emergency.

Drug and Over-the-Counter Remedy Interactions

Herbs and dietary supplements are sometimes helpful for patients. Some natural substances like turmeric, ginger, rosemary, cat's claw, devil's claw, and willow bark are thought to mimic the effects of NSAIDs. They can also lead to the same side effects as NSAIDs, such as GI upset and bleeding.

- *Turmeric* - Many believe that turmeric has cancer fighting, anti-inflammatory and blood thinning properties. The active ingredient in turmeric, curcumin, decreases the levels of two enzymes that cause inflammation. It is sometimes used to fight joint inflammation, for skin disorders, for cancer fighting actions, for the pain associated with sprains and for digestive disorders. Turmeric sold in grocery stores can be simply sprinkled on food; supplemental preparations of turmeric are sold in health food stores.

- *Ginger* - Ginger has been used for thousands of years to treat inflammation, nausea, headaches, menstrual pain and muscular soreness. Ginger root can be added to foods, used as a compress for pain when the root is grated, boiled and then placed on the affected area, and made into a tea.

- *Valerian Root* - Valerian, can be used for pain reduction, stress, anxiety, tension and insomnia. Valerian is believed to decrease the sensitivity of the nerves. Valerian can also be made into a tea.

- *Eucommia* - The bark and leaves of the eucommia plant are used for joint pain, particularly back pain and/or pain in the knees and hips; it is also believed to heal injured tissue and to make tendons, ligaments and bones stronger. Recent research suggests that eucommia contains a substance that promotes the development and growth of collagen. Patients should consult with their doctor, however, before taking eucommia, particularly when they are taking antihypertensive medications.

- *Fish oil* - Current research indicates that fish oil is helpful for treating many diseases and disorders such as asthma, headaches, back pain, depression, cardiovascular problems, rheumatoid arthritis, neurological pain, and chronic inflammation. The recommended dose is 2-4 grams of DHA + EPA daily. Fish oil omega-3 fatty acids are often combined with other agents such as turmeric and ginger to potentiate its pain relief effects.

- *Vitamin D* - Vitamin D supplementation may be beneficial for chronic pain because research studies have found that low levels of vitamin D are associated with increased levels of chronic pain.

Medications can interact with a number of things. Some interactions include those with other medications including over-the-counter drugs, foods, and lifestyle choices, such as alcohol use, herbs and other natural substances. Some of these interactions are synergistic and others impede the action of the medication.

Substance Abuse

Substance abuse is defined as the overindulgence or dependence on an addictive substance, usually alcohol or illegal drugs. As with the abuse of some types of illegal drugs, withdrawal occurs when a chronic user of alcohol suddenly stops drinking.

Signs and Symptoms

Chronic alcohol abuse is drinking on a regular basis to a point of intoxication or drinking to the level of intoxication on a continuous basis. Chronic alcohol abuse can cause health problems and problems of other natures. Chronic drug abuse is defined as the habitual abuse of drugs to the extent that the abuse significantly injures the user by way of physical, social or economic harm. Anyone who becomes unable to control their use of drugs, even after they have been harmed by the use, is considered a chronic drug abuser.

Drug-seeking behavior is a pattern of behavior in which a person tries to obtain prescription medications, such as narcotic pain, anxiety or tranquilizers. Some examples of this are false identification, forged or adjusted prescriptions, repeated requests for refills of "lost" or "stolen" medication, falsely reporting pain or anxiety, and abusive or threatening behavior when denied medications

Nurses, physicians and pharmacists must be able to identify drug-seeking behavior.

Shock

Simply stated, shock is a condition where body tissue is not sufficiently perfused; the oxygen demands exceed the amount of oxygen available to the body.

The four stages of shock are:

1. *Initial Stage* - Hypoxia occurs as the result of hypoperfusion. Lactic acid rises during this stage because of oxygen deprivation.

2. *Compensatory Stage* - The body attempts to reverse the condition by using certain compensatory, physiological mechanisms. Hyperventilation attempts to blow off the increasing carbon dioxide and raise the blood pH. Epinephrine and norepinephrine are released into the body by the arterial baroreceptors. Epinephrine causes the heart rate to increase and norepinephrine increases the heart rate and may lead to vasoconstriction. Anti-diuretic hormone (ADH) is also released to save the kidneys with vasopressin.

3. *Progressive Stage* - Compensatory mechanisms begin to fail. Sodium ions build up, potassium ions leak out, metabolic acidosis increases, blood remains in the capillaries, histamine is released, fluid and proteins leak into surrounding tissues, the blood thickens and vital bodily organs are severely threatened.

4. *Refractory Stage or Final Stage* – At this stage, shock can no longer be reversed and death is imminent.

Cardiogenic Shock

This form of shock occurs when the ventricles of the heart are not functioning properly; this malfunction leads to inadequate circulation and reduced cardiac output. The most common cause of cardiogenic shock is myocardial muscle damage secondary to a serious myocardial infarction. Some of the other causes are heart failure, cardiac valve problems, dysrhythmias, cardiomyopathy and myocarditis.

Signs and Symptoms

Cardiogenic shock's signs and symptoms include peripheral vasoconstriction, which limits blood flow to vital organs like the heart and the brain, as well as hypotension, tachycardia, oliguria and lethargy.

Anaphylactic Shock

This type of distributive shock occurs when the body's immune system over reacts with systemic circulatory relaxation. Anaphylactic shock most often occurs as the result of an allergic response to a medication, such as penicillin.

Signs and Symptoms

The signs and symptoms include massive relaxation of the blood vessels, decreased cardiac output, histamine release, a drop in blood pressure, pooling of venous blood, laryngeal edema, a rash, and a rapid, pounding heartbeat.

Treatment

If the cause of the anaphylaxis is an IV antibiotic, the IV must be immediately removed. Adrenaline or noradrenaline is also given to reduce laryngeal edema and to constrict the vasculature.

Neurogenic Shock

Neurogenic shock results when the sympathetic nervous system shuts down. It is most often associated with blocked spinal nerve functioning secondary to a spinal cord injury or during the administration of a spinal anesthetic.

Signs and Symptoms

The arterioles and venules are relaxed. Bradycardia, hypotension, syncope and fainting can occur.

Treatment

The treatment aims to remove and correct the underlying cause. Intravenous sympathetic stimulation medications like atropine or metaraminol are administered.

Septic Shock

Septic shock is a systemic, multisystem response to a serious infection; it is associated with a high incidence of morbidity and mortality. Some of the risk factors for septic shock include a surgical or invasive procedure infection, immunocompromise, leukemia, and lymphoma. The most common pathogens are gram-positive bacteria, like *staphylococcus aureus* and *streptococcus pneumoniae*, gram-negative bacteria, such as *Escherichia coli* and *pseudomonas aeruginosa*, and other microorganisms such as a virus, fungus and parasites.

Some of the ways that infections, bacteremia, sepsis and septic shock can be prevented are to minimize the use of invasive procedures and treatments to the greatest extent possible. All invasive procedures, like surgery, endoscopy, and all invasive treatments, like central lines, intravenous lines, and urinary catheters place patients at risk for an infection.

Signs and Symptoms

Massive vasodilation, cardiac depression, the formation of microemboli, and the abnormal distribution of intravascular fluid occur.

Early signs and symptoms include hypotension, flushed, warm skin, a widened pulse pressure, tachycardia, hyperventilation, metabolic acidosis, respiratory alkalosis, adventitious breath sounds like crackles, hypoxia, pulmonary edema, confusion and lethargy; late signs include highly serious decreases in cardiac output, peripheral vasoconstriction, and life threatening hypoxia that affects virtually all bodily systems.

Signs and symptoms of infection, such as a fever and an elevated white blood cell count accompanied by hypotension, indicate the presence of septic shock.

Hypotension accompanied by a bounding pulse is often the key clinical manifestation of sepsis.

Treatment

Fluids are administered to restore fluid that has left the vascular spaces and to correct for the peripheral vasodilation. Other treatments can include mechanical ventilation, oxygen supplementation, possible dialysis, and medications including antibiotics for the infection, vasopressors such as noradrenaline medications to increase the blood pressure and ongoing hemodynamic monitoring.

Hypovolemic Shock

The stages of hypovolemic shock range from 1 to 4; stage 1 has minimal signs and symptoms and little blood loss; and stage 4 is characterized by severe clinical signs and symptoms, and large blood losses greater than 40% of the patient's total circulating volume.

Hypovolemic shock is the most common type of shock. Primary, hypovolemic shock results from hemorrhage or the loss of fluid from the body's circulatory system. Patients are at risk of this type of shock, are those who suffer from burns, extreme dehydration, diabetic ketoacidosis, diabetes insipidus and those who have been exposed to environmental hazards.

Signs and Symptoms

The signs and symptoms that a patient may experience due to hypovolemic shock include pale skin, oral dryness, poor skin turgor and excessive thirst, which is a sign of dehydration, and due to diminished circulating hemoglobin, tachypnea can also occur.

1. *Initial Stage*: Hypoxia occurs as the result of hypoperfusion.

2. *Compensatory Stage*: Compensatory mechanisms such as hyperventilation (to raise PH and decrease carbon dioxide levels), decreased cardiac output (vasodilation), tachycardia (norepinephrine and epinephrine release), and diminished urinary output (anti-diuretic hormone release to protect the kidneys with vasopressin).

3. *Progressive Stage*: Metabolic acidosis, increased blood viscosity with accompanying impaired microcirculation, which severely compromises the perfusion of all vital organs (Multisystem failure).

4. *Refractory or Irreversible Stage*: Vital organs have failed; death is imminent.

Treatment

Ongoing assessments and the immediate correction of the cause (bleeding, dehydration) and the replacement of blood and fluid volume are necessary to preserve life. Hypovolemic shock is a life-threatening event. Multiple intravenous catheters are placed and fluids like Lactated Ringers are administered at a rapid rate as well as blood, blood components and plasma expanders, as indicated.

Obstructive Shock

Obstructive shock occurs when there is an obstruction of the flow of blood outside of the heart into a major vessel, such as occurs when an embolus enters a major vessel. Obstructive shock, unlike other forms of shock, can affect relatively healthy people without any traumatic injury.

Like other forms of shock, the protective, compensatory baroreceptor reflexes protect the body's most essential organs at the expense of other bodily organs.

Signs and Symptoms

The signs and symptoms of obstructive shock include oliguria hypotension, tachycardia, and cyanosis.

Treatment

The goal of treatment is to identify and correct the underlying cause such as a tension pneumothorax, aortic stenosis, cardiac tamponade or pulmonary embolism.

Allergic Reactions

Allergic reactions, a hypersensitive immune response, can occur from medications, foods and environmental sources. Some are minor and others, such as anaphylaxis which was discussed previously, can be very serious and life threatening.

Signs and Symptoms

The signs and symptoms vary according to the antigen and the method of contact. Some commonly occurring signs and symptoms include coughing, dyspnea, wheezing, a rash, swelling and itchiness.

Treatment

Treatments, including prevention, can include an antihistamine, a corticosteroid cream for affected skin and itchiness, and epinephrine for severe allergic responses.

Blood Dyscrasia

Blood dyscrasia is a blood disorder in which one part of the blood does not manifest in the normal supply. This disorder generally appears when red blood cell, white blood cell, or platelet counts are overly elevated or diminished. Types of blood dyscrasias include:

- Von Willebrand's disease, blood clotting as a result of low protein supply

- Hemophilia, which occurs due to blood clotting diseases

- Thrombocytopenia, which is a low platelet count resulting in decrease of platelet production and excessive bleeding

- Anemia or low red blood cells

Signs and Symptoms

General signs and symptoms include decrease in red blood cells, wan appearance, weakness, and higher infection rate resulting from decrease in white blood cells. Blood dyscrasias may also be induced by specific diseases. Symptoms of these include idiopathic thrombocytopenic purpura, causing sudden small and large bleeding points on the skin; thrombotic thrombocytopenic purpura, causing bleeding and anemia; Von Willebrand disorder, causing bleeding gums and nose bleeds; and hemophilia, causing bleeding in the joints and facilitating bruising.

Treatment

Treatment includes medicines, chemotherapy, and transfusion of blood products and bone marrow transplants at times. Other helpful treatments include steroids, and the replacement of red or white blood cells as indicated.

Disseminated Intravascular Coagulation (DIC)

This disorder occurs because of several underlying conditions and diseases. It does not occur as a primary condition; it is always secondary to some other condition or disease. This disorder is somewhat paradoxical. It affects thrombosis, or clotting, as well as bleeding. There is a lack of balance between anticoagulation and coagulation.

Signs and Symptoms

The chronic form of disseminated intravascular coagulation has a slow onset over weeks or months and it leads to excessive clotting without bleeding. Acute DIC occurs rapidly and is marked by excessive clotting and then severe bleeding. Other signs and symptoms can include headache, tachycardia, hypotension, changes in mood, behavior and/or level of consciousness, and peripheral cyanosis secondary to microvascular thrombosis.

Treatment

Non-pharmacological and pharmacological interventions aim to prevent life threatening complications, such as impaired perfusion and death, to maintain tissue and organ perfusion and to eliminate the root cause, if possible. Specific interventions include the administration of blood products like packed red cells, and fresh frozen plasma to replace clotting factors and fluids. Hypoxia, acidosis, and hypotension are corrected and recombinant human activated protein C may be administered.

Electrolyte/Fluid Imbalances

Electrolyte imbalances are an inadequate balance of the electrolytes, which include potassium, calcium, magnesium and sodium, in the bloodstream.

Signs and Symptoms

There is a variety of symptoms associated with electrolyte imbalances. They can accompany other symptoms, which can vary depending on the underlying disease or disorder. The general symptoms that may occur with an electrolyte imbalance include fatigue, nausea without vomiting, dizziness, trembling, constipation, dark urine, decreased urine output, muscle weakness, stiff or aching joints, dry skin, dry mouth, and bad breath. Serious symptoms are poor elasticity of the skin, tachycardia, sunken eyes, and a change in mental status, such as confusion, delirium, hallucinations or delusions.

Treatment

Treatment of electrolyte imbalances is dependent on what type of electrolyte is actually affected. For example, a patient with low potassium levels should be urged to watch their diet, take potassium supplements and be given intravenous treatments. If a patient's potassium levels are high, the treatment is diuretics and potassium given intravenously.

In addition to the immediate treatment for the imbalance, it is vital that the cause for the imbalance is discovered and corrected. Possible causes include kidney disease, hormone/endocrine problems, stomach disorders, improper diet, loss of bodily fluids due to illness and the side effects of chemotherapy or medications. Some types of medications that can cause an electrolyte imbalance in the body are steroids, tricyclic antidepressants, birth control pills, diuretics, cough medicines, laxatives, steroids and excessive use of antacids.

Adrenal Insufficiency: Addison's Disease

Addison's disease is a chronic adrenocortical insufficiency, caused by a primary deficiency of the adrenal cortex. It occurs primarily among women and adults under the age of sixty, but it can occur at any age. It is also associated with cancer, tuberculosis or AIDS, which affects the adrenal glands.

Signs and Symptoms

This disorder has a primary and secondary form. The primary form is marked by hyperkalemia, hypotension, hyponatremia, darkened skin pigmentation, insufficient mineralocorticoid levels, dehydration, renal failure, shock and death. Secondary adrenal insufficiency is NOT characterized by insufficient mineralocorticoid levels, but there is a slight hyperpigmentation and a mild degree of water retention and low serum sodium levels secondary to this retention. Other signs and symptoms include fatigue, muscular aches, hypoglycemia, weight loss, confusion, nausea, vomiting, anorexia, diarrhea, menstrual changes, tremors and joint pain.

Treatment

Intravenous fluids, steroids, and rest are used for adrenal crisis; hydrocortisone, prednisone, prednisolone, methylprednisolone or dexamethasone are used to treat primary and secondary cortisol deficiency. The most serious complication of Addison's disease is adrenal hemorrhage septicemia, which is treated by aggressive antibiotic therapy, intravenous vasopressors and large doses of steroids.

Hypercortisolism

Cushing's syndrome is a chronic hyper-secretion of glucocorticoids from the adrenal cortex. It is most common in women 30-50 years old, and patients with a pituitary tumor are also at a higher risk, especially if they take steroids, as often occurs after an organ transplant, or when steroids are used adjunct to chemotherapy.

Signs and Symptoms

This disorder affects many bodily functions because the metabolism of proteins, carbohydrates and fats is altered. Altered carbohydrate metabolism is characterized by hyperglycemia secondary to impaired insulin utilization, and hepatic gluconeogenesis. Some of these signs and symptoms include muscular weakness and wasting, osteoporosis, bone pain, pathological fractures, purple striae, thin, fragile skin and bruising related to the loss of collagen as the result of altered protein metabolism. Altered fat metabolism can result in a moon face, buffalo hump of the back and a pendulous abdomen. Other signs and symptoms include compromised Inflammatory and immune responses which places the person at risk for serious infections, acne, Oligomenorrhea, amenorrhea, excessive androgen which can lead to hirsutism, impotence and libido changes, altered water and mineral metabolism as characterized by hypertension, hypochloremia, weight gain, edema, metabolic alkalosis, osteoporosis, and increased calcium reabsorption. Hematological changes may also occur, including high red blood cell counts, increased hematocrit and hemoglobin, leukocytosis, eosinopenia and lymphopenia. Mental and emotional responses, such as psychosis, emotional instability, anxiety, depression, and memory losses may occur.

Treatment

Surgical interventions include an adrenalectomy, removal of an adrenal cortex tumor, and a hypophysectomy to remove a pituitary tumor when this is the cause. Stereotactic irradiation is also performed on patients who have a small adenoma; medications can include mitotane, aminoglutethemide or metyrapone.

Aldosteronism

Primary aldosteronism is most often found among women and it is often associated with adrenal hyperplasia; secondary aldosteronism can be caused by pregnancy and renal artery stenosis.

Signs and Symptoms

These include low renin, hypertension, hypokalemia and resulting muscle weakness.

Treatment

When a mass, or tumor, is not present and surgically removable, the patient is treated with medications such as spironolactone, amiloride or eplerenone, sodium intake restriction of less than 100 meq/day, weight control, exercise and the avoidance of alcohol. The interventions prevent resulting hypertension.

Pheochromocytoma: Adrenal Medulla Hypersecretion

Pheochromocytoma is a disorder in which the adrenal medulla hyper-secretes catecholamines, primarily norepinephrine. It typically affects those between the ages of 40 and 60. Pheochromocytoma is primarily caused by adrenal gland tumors, although some cases result from extra-adrenal tumors.

Signs and Symptoms

This disorder is characterized by the five Ps of pallor, palpitations, profuse perspiration, pain (chest, abdominal and headache pain), and pressure (high blood pressure). Other signs and symptoms include tremors, weight loss, constipation, orthostatic hypotension, hyperglycemia, retinopathy and hypercalcemia.

Treatment

Surgical treatment includes the removal of the adrenal and/or extra adrenal pheochromocytoma after which catecholamine blockage is achieved with an alpha-adrenergic blocker (phenoxybenzamine) followed by a beta-adrenergic blocker. At times, a calcium channel blocker is helpful.

Hypoglycemia

Extremely low blood glucose level, or hypoglycemia, is usually associated with diabetics who have exercised excessively, had too much insulin or too little food.

Signs and Symptoms

Signs and symptoms of hypoglycemia include excessive hunger, sweating, anxiety, shakiness, heart palpitations, double or blurry vision, and confusion. Uncommon symptoms include loss of consciousness, seizures, coma and death. Left untreated, the person will lose brain functioning.

Treatment

The treatment of hypoglycemia is the immediate ingestion of candy, fruit juice, glucose or glucose tablets when the patient is conscious; intravenous glucose is used when the patient is unconscious and/or not responded to given oral interventions.

Hyperglycemia

Hyperglycemia, or high blood glucose, is defined as a fasting (8-hour) blood glucose level greater than 180 mg/dL. Unlike hypoglycemia, hyperglycemia leads to long-term adverse effects but it is not usually life-threatening.

Signs and Symptoms

Early signs and symptoms include fatigue, blurred vision, excessive thirst, headache, and frequent urination. If these are left untreated, hyperosmolar syndrome can occur and ketones build up in the blood and urine (ketoacidosis).

If hyperglycemia is left untreated, there are several potential long-term complications. These complications include renal failure, nephropathy, diabetic retinopathy, bone and joint problems such as osteoporosis, skin problems, including bacterial infections, fungal infections and non-healing wounds, chronic infections, oral tooth and gum infections, cataracts, cardiovascular disease, stroke, neuropathy, and foot disorders including infections, necrosis, and impaired blood flow.

Treatment

Hyperglycemia is treated with the administration of insulin. It can be prevented with a specific diabetes meal plan, monitoring blood glucose levels and medications, which may require adjustments for overeating and the lack of physical activity.

Diabetic Ketoacidosis

Diabetic ketoacidosis occurs as the result of severe hyperglycemia.

Signs and Symptoms

The signs and symptoms of diabetic ketoacidosis usually develop rapidly and include nausea and vomiting, abdominal pain, confusion, excessive thirst, weakness or fatigue, shortness of breath, fruity-scented breath and frequent urination.

Treatment

Patients diagnosed with diabetic ketoacidosis may be treated in the emergency department or they may have to be admitted to the hospital for treatment. Treatment includes a three-step process, which includes rehydration, replacement of electrolytes like sodium, chloride and potassium, and intravenous insulin therapy until blood glucose is less than 240 mg/dL and no longer acidic. If diabetic ketoacidosis is left untreated, it can lead to unconsciousness and even death.

Hyperglycemic Hyperosmolar Non-ketotic Syndrome (HHNS)

HHNS is a condition that occurs due to infections, and in diabetics and the elderly.

Signs and Symptoms

Some of the early signs and symptoms of HHNS include lethargy, nausea, weight loss, coma, fever, convulsions, confusion, weakness, increased thirst, and increased urination. Later signs and symptoms include speech alterations, loss of feeling or function of one's muscles, seizures, coma and eventually death.

Treatment

This includes intravenous fluids with potassium, intravenous insulin and other supportive medications to correct the patient's blood pressure, urinary output, level of hydration and/or circulation problems.

Hyperthyroidism: Grave's Disease and Thyrotoxicosis

Thyrotoxicosis and Graves's disease account for the vast majority of hyperthyroidism. Grave's disease is associated with an autoimmune disorder like myasthenia gravis, genetics, trauma, infections, thyroid cancer, thyroid-stimulating hormone-secreting pituitary adenomas and medications like amiodarone. Severe hyperthyroidism can cause a thyroid storm or crisis, a life-threatening condition with a high mortality rate.

Signs and Symptoms

The signs and symptoms are dangerously high blood pressure, fever, pronounced tachycardia, respiratory distress, and severe tachycardia when thyroid storm occurs.

Less severe cases of hyperthyroidism are characterized by warm skin, hyper-metabolism, exophthalmos (bulging eyeballs), fine hair, alopecia, heat intolerance, increased diaphoresis, insomnia, anxiety, muscular weakness and diarrhea.

Treatment

Emergency treatments include the stabilization of the cardiovascular and respiratory status, the reduction of thyroid hormone secretion and synthesis, fluids, glucose and other electrolyte replacements, as well as the reduction of fever without the use of aspirin, which can increase the amount of free thyroid hormone. Medications include methimazole, propylthiourcil and radioiodine. Increased dietary calories and nutrients help, as can the surgical removal of the thyroid gland.

Hypothyroidism

This endocrine disorder can result from primary, secondary and tertiary thyroid failures such as occurs with Hashimoto's disease, a thyroid stimulating hormone deficiency and deficient thyrotropin releasing hormone, respectively. Hashimoto's disease is the most common cause of hypothyroidism in the United States. Other risk factors are neck radiation therapy, diabetes, Addison's disease, pernicious anemia, amiodarone and/or lithium therapy and/or a family history of thyroid disease.

Signs and Symptoms

The many signs and symptoms of hypothyroidism include decreased T3 and T4 levels accompanied by elevated TSH levels constipation, hoarseness of the voice, pallor, dry skin, stiff muscles, edema, anorexia, weight gain, menstrual alterations, bradycardia, cardiac enlargement and anemia.

The most serious of all complications is myxedema coma, a severe case of hypothyroidism, which presents with coma, respiratory failure, cardiac failure, decreased cardiac output, edema, especially around the feet, eyes and hands, adrenal insufficiency, severe hypothermia, and other signs of severe hypothyroidism.

Treatment

The replacement of the thyroid hormone is the primary treatment; a subtotal thyroidectomy may be necessary for large goiters.

Myxedema coma mandates the immediate intravenous administration of levothyroxine sodium, glucose and corticosteroids. At times, intubation, mechanical ventilation and cardiovascular support are indicated.

Hemophilia

Hemophilia is a hereditary recessive genetic disorder that leads to a deficiency in clotting factor VIII (hemophilia A) or clotting IX (hemophilia B). Types A and B only affect males. There is a less common C-type that can affect females.

Signs and Symptoms

The primary signs and symptoms include internal or external bleeding with a prolonged partial thromboplastin with normal bleeding, prothrombin, and thrombin times, joint bleeding, joint deformity and permanent disfigurement and dysfunction. C cerebral hemorrhage can lead to increased intracranial pressure and death.

Treatment

Hemophilia is treated with infusions of deficient clotting factors, Advate, Xyntha (an anti-hemophilic factor) Kogenate and gene therapy. Some of these treatments are preventive and others are used for emergency treatment.

HIV/AIDS

People all over the globe are affected with this syndrome. It is considered a blood-borne sexually transmitted disease, although it can also be spread by non-sexual contact with bodily fluids. Healthcare workers are at risk for occupational exposures to HIV and other risk factors include unsafe sexual practices, intravenous drug use and perinatal exposure during pregnancy.

Signs and Symptoms

HIV infections can range from asymptomatic primary infections to AIDS, which is often complicated with opportunistic infections that can lead to death. These infections can affect the pulmonary system (pneumocystis carinii pneumonia), the nervous system (blindness, peripheral neuropathy), the musculoskeletal system (arthralgia, wasting and weakness) and they can also include Kaposi's sarcoma, mycobacterium avium infections, candidiasis, cytomegalovirus which affects the gastrointestinal tract, herpes simplex, histoplasmosis, salmonella, toxoplasma gondii, tuberculosis, acid-base imbalances and fluid and electrolyte disorders.

Some of the signs and symptoms associated with this infection include chills, diarrhea, oral lesions, abdominal discomfort, weight loss, fever, night sweats, dry cough, dyspnea, lethargy, malaise, skin rash, headaches, lymphadenopathy, progressive edema, stiff neck, confusion and seizures.

Treatment

Highly active combination antiretroviral therapy (HAART) decreases the viral load, increases the CD4 T-cells and prevents secondary opportunistic infections and cancers. These medications include nucleoside reverse transcriptase inhibitors (Zidovudine), nonnucleoside reverse transcriptase inhibitors (Efavirenz), protease inhibitors (Lopinavir and Ritonavir, fusion inhibitors and combination antiretroviral agents (Combivir and Trizivir). Patients with HIV/AIDS at the ER often have an infection. Treatments vary according to the patient's symptoms and infection.

Acute Renal Failure

Renal failure can be acute or chronic. Acute renal failure can be caused by a circulatory deficiency to the kidney, which can occur secondary to an infection, a drop in blood pressure, hemorrhage and inadequate hydration. It can also result from renal obstructions, some medications like gentamicin, streptomycin, naproxen and ACE inhibitors, as well as poisoning.

Signs and Symptoms

The signs and symptoms of acute renal failure include oliguria, anuria, edema, anorexia, nausea, vomiting, confusion, anxiety and flank pain.

Treatment

The treatment of acute and chronic renal failure is discussed below.

Chronic Renal Failure

Chronic renal failure is characterized by minimum renal functioning. It sometimes occurs with end-stage renal disease, but most often occurs as the result of long standing disease such as diabetes, hypertension and untreated acute renal failure. Other less common disorders that pose the risk of chronic renal failure include exposures to toxic chemicals, some autoimmune disorders like systemic lupus erythematosus, congenital renal abnormalities, trauma and infection.

Signs and Symptoms

Early signs and symptoms include anorexia, fatigue, pruritus, dry skin, nausea and weight loss. Later signs and symptoms include hypertension, bone pain, confusion, skin color changes, vomiting extremity numbness, thirst, cramping, numbness, amenorrhea, easy bruising and bleeding, shortness of breath, insomnia, severe edema and restless leg syndrome.

Treatment

Antihypertensive medications are used hypertension causes the renal compromise; diabetes must be controlled and managed to prevent further renal damage. Treatments include hemodialysis, peritoneal dialysis and kidney transplantation, as well as phosphate binders, fluid restrictions, blood transfusions and the treatment of anemia with iron and medications like erythropoietin.

Sickle Cell Anemia/Crisis

Sickle cell anemia is an autosomal recessive genetic disorder that adversely affects hemoglobin in the red blood cells. This disorder can adversely affect virtually all bodily systems. The abnormal sickled cells hemolyze and rupture.

Signs and Symptoms

Among the many signs and symptoms are pain, extreme fatigue, leg ulcerations, ocular damage, bone infarcts and aseptic necrosis, hand and feet swelling (dactylitis), splenic sequestration, anemia, cardiac and pulmonary damage.

Treatment

Pain is relieved with analgesics, heat, fluids and rest; oxygen helps respiratory compromise; hydroxyurea promotes the production of fetal hemoglobin and blood transfusions are given in organ compromise.

Communicable Diseases

Clostridium Difficile (C. Difficile)

C. difficile causes colitis by producing toxins that damage the lining of the colon. It is a relatively common nosocomial infection; however, severe infections can be life threatening, particularly among those with serious disease and immune-compromise.

Signs and Symptoms

These include colitis, abdominal pain and cramping, profuse diarrhea and fever. Serious complications include colon rupture, severe dehydration, and the spread of the infection to the abdominal cavity, thus causing peritonitis and possible sepsis.

Treatment

Antibiotics such as vancomycin and metronidazole are used for treatment; however, recurring cases are much more difficult to treat than a single episode.

Rubeola (Measles)

The rubeola virus is transmitted via airborne or contact with droplets of infectious material from respiratory tract secretions, blood, or urine. It is communicable from 4-5 days prior to emergence of the rash. The incubation period is from 8-20 days.

Signs and Symptoms

These include fever, Koplik spots (a maculopapular, erythematous rash that starts on the face and spreads to the body) followed by desquamation, malaise, coryza, cough and conjunctivitis. Complications include pneumonia, otitis media, bronchiolitis, obstructive laryngitis and encephalitis.

Treatment

Like many other childhood communicable diseases, rubeola treatment is typically supportive with the provision of fluids, fever control, the provision of a darkened room for photophobia, bed rest and isolation until after the fifth day following the appearance of the rash.

Rubella (German Measles)

The rubella virus is transmitted by airborne droplets, and direct and indirect contact with nasopharyngeal secretions, urine or fecal material. The incubation period lasts 14-21 days; it is communicable from 5-7 days before the appearance of the rash.

Signs and Symptoms

These include fever, lymphadenopathy, sore throat, coughing, headache, malaise, coryza, and a rash that appears initially on the face and spreads in a downward manner to the neck, shoulders, trunk and legs. Later, it disappears in an upward manner. The complications include arthritis (in rare cases,) encephalitis and purpura. The greatest danger is rubella's teratogenic effects on a developing fetus.

Treatment

The treatment is supportive, including comfort and isolation for pregnant women.

Varicella

Varicella, or chickenpox, is caused by the herpes varicella-zoster virus. The incubation period ranges from 14-21 days; it is communicable one day before the appearance of the rash and up to six days after the vesicles have formed and crusted over. It is transmitted by direct contact, droplets and contaminated objects known as fomites.

Signs and Symptoms

Anorexia, fever, malaise, a highly itchy rash on the trunk and scalp, and oral/perineal lesions are some of the signs and symptoms of varicella.

Treatment

Some of the interventions for this communicable disease include isolation, supportive care, skin care (topical calamine lotion), and keeping fingernails short or gloved to prevent scratching.

Mumps

Mumps is transmitted with direct contact or droplet transmission of the paramyxovirus; the incubation period ranges from 14-21 days.

Signs and Symptoms

Malaise, fever, headache, anorexia, earache and parotid gland swelling.

Treatment

The treatment is supportive and symptomatic.

Pertussis (Whooping Cough)

Bordetella pertussis is transmitted by respiratory droplets and direct contact. Whooping cough is transmissible from seven days after initial exposure through three weeks after the coughing has begun. period ranges from 3-12 days after exposure.

Signs and Symptoms

The signs and symptoms vary according to the phase, or stage, of this infectious disease, as follows:

1. *Catarrhal Stage* - Increased lacrimation, a mild cough, rhinorrhea, conjunctivitis, and a low grade fever

2. *Paroxysmal Stage* - Vomiting, malaise, fatigue, severe coughing leading to cyanosis and exhaustion

3. *Convalescent Stage* - Coughing subsides

Treatment

Bed rest, a quiet environment, increased fluid intake, the administration of erythromycin estolate, azithromycin, or clarithromycin and respiratory suctioning and supplemental oxygen, as indicated.

Diphtheria

Diphtheria can be prevented with a vaccination. It is a respiratory infection caused by the corynebacterium diphtheria. If untreated, it can cause death.

Signs and Symptoms

The signs and symptoms of this infectious disease include malaise, fever, chills, sore throat, coughing, headache, dysphagia, dyspnea, tachypnea, lymphadenopathy, facial paralysis, myocarditis, cardiac arrhythmias, and the presence of a pseudo-membrane on the pharynx, tonsils or nasal passages as well as the skin in less severe cases.

Treatment

Intubation and mechanical ventilation can treat respiratory problems. Cardiac dysrhythmias are also corrected; diphtheria antitoxin will treat respiratory paralysis.

Herpes Zoster (Shingles)

Herpes zoster occurs as the result of the reactivation of the varicella zoster, or chickenpox, virus. The elderly and patients with compromised immunity (or who are taking immunosuppressive drugs) are at greatest risk for shingles. Caucasians contract the disease most often, and females contract it more often than males.

Signs and Symptoms

It is typically characterized by painful thoracic area skin eruptions that don't usually cross the midline. Dermatome(s) are sometimes found in other parts of the body.

Treatment

Vaccines and antiviral medications can lessen the severity and duration.

Mononucleosis

Mononucleosis, also known as the "kissing disease", is caused by the Epstein-Barr virus. The highest incidence is between 15-30 years of age. It is usually self-limiting, with complete recovery after 2-3 weeks.

Signs and Symptoms

Fever, fatigue, malaise, sore throat, headache, aches and pains, spleen enlargement and lymphadenopathy. Rare manifestations include encephalitis and spleen rupture.

Treatment

This infection is treated supportively and symptomatically. Antibiotics are given for secondary strep throats, and NSAIDs are used for aches, pains and fever. The patient should avoid contact sports while their spleen is enlarged.

Respiratory Syncytial Virus (RSV)

RSV commonly causes bronchiolitis, and can lead to respiratory failure.

Signs and Symptoms

Thick mucus that occludes the bronchioles, coughing, respiratory stridor, wheezing, tachypnea, cyanosis, listlessness, pharyngitis, Hypercapnia and apneic spell.

Treatment

The treatment of RSV includes supportive care, symptom management and antibiotics if a bacterial infection is suspected. Intravenous hydration, supplemental O2 administration, and respiratory interventions are provided as indicated.

Meningitis

Meningitis is an inflammation of the pia layers of the meninges and the cerebrospinal fluid which can be caused by a number of viruses, bacteria and fungi including *haemophilius influenzae, streptococcus pneumoniae*, group B streptococcus, *neisseria meningitidis, E. coli*, serratia and enterobacter. Meningitis can be life-threatening.

Signs and Symptoms

These include stiff neck, fever, headache, altered mental status, petechial or purpural rash, arching of the back & neck, blank staring, seizures, photophobia, positive Brudzinski's and Kernig's signs and bulging fontanels among infants.

Encephalitis

Encephalitis, an inflammation of cerebral tissue, is most often accompanied by meningeal inflammation from a virus. Acute viral encephalitis can be caused by herpes simplex, the West Nile virus, and toxoplasma; adults may be affected with post-ischemic inflammatory encephalitis following a cerebrovascular accident.

Signs and Symptoms

These include nausea, vomiting, fever, headache, altered neurological functioning, motor weakness, disorientation, seizures and unusual behavioral changes.

Treatment

Interventions include the prevention of injury with seizure precautions, maintaining quiet, medications as prescribed, assessing and monitoring neurological status frequently, reorienting the person, monitoring of the vital signs and administering antipyretics and intravenous fluids as needed.

Multi-Drug Resistant Organisms

Standard and transmission-based precautions are necessary to prevent the spread of infections, particularly since there are many resistant strains of microorganisms. Some of these are methicillin-resistant *staphylococcus aureus* (MRSA), vancomycin-resistant *enterococcus* (VRE) and penicillin-resistant *streptococcus pneumoniae*.

Tuberculosis (TB)

TB is transmitted by inhalation of the *tubercle bacilli*. This inflammatory process and its cellular reactions create a firm, small, white nodule called a primary tubercle, the center of which contains the bacilli. Negative air pressure rooms and HEPA masks prevent nosocomial transmission. The disease can lay dormant for years and cause no ill effects. Then, when under some type of physical or emotional stress, the bacilli start to multiply, causing destruction of lung tissue and resulting in mortality. Immunocompromised patients, such as those with HIV/AIDS, are at risk for TB.

Signs and Symptoms

The clinical signs and symptoms of TB include pallor, fever, chills, night sweats, anorexia, productive, purulent cough that can be bloody, dyspnea, chest pain and easy fatigability. The most threatening complication of TB is the development of an untreatable, drug-resistant strain of TB.

Treatment

A combination of medications is the most effective form of treatment - options include INH, rifampin, rifabutin, rifapentine, pyrazinamide, ethambutol, streptomycin, capreomycin, aminosalicylate sodium, cycloserine and ethionamide.

Section 2: Professional Issues

Fundamentals of Nursing

Critical Incident Stress Management

Emergency department nurses work in extremely stressful environments and they are often witness to horrific injuries and accidents, all of which can adversely affect their level of functioning. Critical incident stress management techniques are often employed to alleviate this stress. Although somewhat similar to posttraumatic stress disorder, critical incident stress is more short-lived. It typically persists for only a couple of days or weeks.

Critical incident stress debriefing can be a group process with a skilled facilitator or it can be a peer supportive group run by and facilitated by nurses. During these sessions, the participants are encouraged to verbalize and express their feelings and reactions to the stressors in an open, honest, caring and supportive environment in order to resolve the stress in a healthy and successful manner.

Ethical Dilemmas

The American Nurses Association's Code of Ethics applies to all nurses, including emergency department nurses, in all diverse roles and in all healthcare settings. This code emphasizes the dignity and worth of all people without discrimination, the nurses' commitment to patients, advocacy, accountability, the preservation of safety, patient rights, such as dignity, autonomy and confidentiality, competency, the provision of quality care, collaboration, the integrity of the nursing profession and the resolution of ethical dilemmas and/or conflicts. Some of the ethical principles that nurses must adhere to during all aspects of nursing care and practice are:

- *Justice* - Justice requires nurses to treat all patients fairly. For example, limited resources must be distributed among patients fairly and justly.

- *Fidelity* – Nurses must remain faithful to their promises. The nature of the nurse-patient relationship implies that nurses keep their professional promises and fulfil their responsibilities by providing patients with the best and safest care possible, in a competent and scientific context, while supporting the choices and rights of the patient.

- *Nonmaleficence* – According to the Hippocratic Oath, nonmaleficence is "do no harm." Harm can be intentional or unintentional, as is the case when a patient has an adverse effect to a medication, such as a chemotherapy drug. For obvious reasons, intentional harm is much more serious than unintentional harm.

- *Beneficence* - Although beneficence may appear to be the opposite of nonmaleficence, it is not. Beneficence, simply stated, means "Do good". Doing "good" is more than just not doing harm). On occasions, beneficence can lead to unanticipated harm. For example, when a nurse administers an ordered medication and it leads to side effects, these side effects are considered an unanticipated side effect or unanticipated harm.

- *Accountability* - Nurses are accountable for all aspects of nursing care. They must answer to themselves, their patients and society for their actions and they must accept, personal and professional consequences for their actions.

- *Autonomy and Self Determination* - Each individual may make choices free from coercion or the undue influence of others. Nurses, including emergency department nurses, must never impose their beliefs, values or opinions on the patient. They accept patient choices without judgments; the patient has the right to choose and/or refuse treatments or interventions.

- *Veracity* - Veracity is truthfulness. Nurses do not withhold the whole truth from patients even when it may be upsetting or distressful.

Ethical dilemmas and conflicts are on the rise because of a number of factors, including the wide variety and diversity of treatment options and the ongoing debate about who should get limited healthcare resources. Nurses must identify sources of ethical conflict and initiate changes to avoid them. Many healthcare facilities have multidisciplinary ethics committees that convene to resolve ethical dilemmas and conflicts. Ideally, the members of this committee have had some advanced training and education relating to bioethics to maximize their ability to provide guidance in respect to ethical dilemmas and conflicts.

Some of the commonly occurring ethical dilemmas that affect patients revolve around physician-assisted suicide, the administration of pain medications to relieve pain even when it hastens death, advance directives and withholding food and fluids.

Evidence-Based Practice (EBP)

EBP is research-based practice. Simply stated, EBP begins with research, which is applied to the development of guidelines disseminated through many channels, including publications and professional conferences. These EBP guidelines can and should be applied after the research and guidelines are critiqued by the nurse.

Some areas of consideration for integrating EBP into one's role as a nurse include:

- Is the EBP feasible and practical?
- Do the potential benefits outweigh the possible risks and costs?
- Is it effective and efficient or too time consuming and limited?

Providing an evidence-based approach to care requires that the nurse:

- Access and appraise evidence (research findings)
- Understand the relationships between research and the strength of evidence
- Determine applicability to a patient's condition, context and wishes.

Research and EBP Databases

Some of the databases that nurses can use to review research and EBP are listed below along with the correlate internet link:

1. The Cochrane Library

    http://www.thecochranelibrary.com/view/0/AboutTheCochraneLibrary.html

2. The Joanna Briggs Institute

    http://www.joannabriggs.edu.au/

3. Ovid's Evidence-based Medicine Reviews (EBMR)

    http://www.ovid.com/webapp/wcs/stores/servlet/ProductDisplay?storeId=13051&catalogId=13151&langId=-1&partNumber=Prod-904410

4. Medlars

    http://www.nlm.nih.gov/bsd/mmshome.html

5. Medline Plus (An International nursing index and Index Medicus is also included)

http://www.nlm.nih.gov/medlineplus/

6. Pub Med

   http://www.ncbi.nlm.nih.gov/pubmed/

7. The Cumulative Index to Nursing and Allied Health Literature (CINAHL)
   http://www.ebscohost.com/cinahl/)

8. The Directory of Open Access Journals (Free)

   http://www.doaj.org

9. The Nursing Center for Lippincott Williams & Wilkins'

   http://nursingcenter.com

Lifelong Learning

Lifelong learning is a professional duty and responsibility. The emergency nurse can use a variety of methods to continue their education and ensure their ongoing competency to practice. Learning activities can include reading professional literature, taking courses online, attending seminars and conferences held by professional organizations and associations as well as reading research studies.

Research

Most people recognize that the nursing profession began with the efforts and contributions of Florence Nightingale during the 1850s. Florence Nightingale also instituted the practice of nurse research by observing, collecting and organizing data. Her first research study led to better sanitation and a reduction in mortality rates among the wounded. Nursing research almost completely stopped after her efforts, primarily because relatively few nurses had advanced academic degrees, and nursing journals were relatively rare. It resumed in earnest in the 1960s.

Now, nursing research, is on an accelerated path. All nurses, whether they know it or not, engage in research every time they participate in a pilot program or study that tests a new procedure or piece of equipment, and each time they collect data or more actively participate in a quality assurance or performance improvement study. They also use findings when they use EBP. Now, virtually all nurses can, and should, engage in research and add to the body of nursing knowledge.

Steps of the Research Process

1. The Research Problem
2. The Purpose
3. The Literature Review
4. The Theoretical Framework or Conceptual Framework
5. The Hypothesis/Research Questions
6. Research Design
7. Sample Type and Size
8. Legal and Ethical Issues
9. Instruments and Measurement Tools
10. Validity and Reliability
11. Data Collection Procedure
12. Data Analysis
13. Results
14. Discussion of Findings
15. Conclusions, Implications, Limitations and Recommendations
16. References
17. Communicating Research Results

Forensic Evidence Collection

Forensic specimens are legal evidence that will, or can be, used during the course of legal proceedings when a crime is committed or suspected. For this reason, the chain of custody and its integrity must be maintained. Evidence must be free of contamination; it should only be touched when necessary and, then, gloves are indicated. Clean gloves are necessary for each and every piece of evidence.

Documentation of this collection must include exactly which piece of evidence was touched with a gloved hand, when it was touched, how it was touched and who touched it.

The chain of evidence, also referred to as the chain of custody, is best ensured when the fewest possible people are involved in the collection and the preservation of the evidence. The chain of evidence supports the usefulness and integrity of the evidence and it ensures that evidence can be used for a police investigation and by a court of law. Thorough documentation of evidence must include who handled the evidence and where it was passed so that the continuity of evidence possession is clear and accurate. All collected evidence should be stored in a safe and secure manner, according to the organization's policies and procedures.

Paper bags, rather than plastic bags, are used for evidence because plastic tends to create moisture, which could destroy or compromise its integrity. All collected evidence should be stored in a safe and secure manner, according to the organization's policies and procedures.

Patient Safety

Falls and Falls Prevention

Falls are one of the most common and most costly patient-related accidents in health care. All patients should be screened and assessed for falls risk upon admission. If the patient is at risk for falls, preventive measures must be implemented.

Some of the risk factors associated with falls include:

- Poor vision

- Slow reaction time

- Incontinence

- Confusion

- Environmental hazards

- Age

- Medications such as sedation

- Poor balance, coordination, gait and range of motion (ROM)

- Past falls

- Fear of falling

- Weak muscles

- Some diseases and disorders like a seizure disorder, a cerebrovascular accident or Parkinson's disease

- Unsafe footwear

- Broken equipment

Preventing falls is a team effort. Special measures and special nursing care must start as soon as any patient or resident is assessed as a falls risk.

Biological Safety: Infection Control and Nosocomial Infections

Most nosocomial infections are spread by the hands of the health care workers from one patient to another. These infections are limited to only those infections that a patient did not have before they were hospitalized, but were acquired after admission or after care was provided. The most commonly occurring risk factors for nosocomial infections are prolonged illness and immunosuppression, treatments such as chemotherapy, invasive procedures like indwelling urinary catheters, and some medications. All equipment and nonsterile supplies can harbor and spread nosocomial infections. They are very costly but are usually preventable.

The urinary tract, the respiratory tract, wounds, and the bloodstream are the most common sites for nosocomial infections; some of the commonly occurring pathogens include *E. coli, Candida albicans, staphylococcus aureus, pseudomonas aeruginosa,* and *enterococcus*.

Hand washing is the single most effective way to prevent nosocomial infections in healthcare facilities. Protective precautions, such as standard precautions and transmission-based precautions, are also necessary, particularly because of the presence of so many resistant strains of pathogens.

Protective precautions include:

- Standard precautions that apply to all blood, bodily fluids and patients regardless of diagnosis

- Contact precautions to prevent direct and indirect contact transmissions, such as with infections contained in diarrhea, wounds, and herpes simplex.

- Precautions for the prevention of airborne microbes like TB. These precautions include a HEPA mask and a negative pressure room.

- Droplet precautions prevent the transmission of pathogens transmitted with a cough or sneeze. Masks are indicated for these precautions.

Oxygen Therapy Safety

A number of precautions need to be taken to allow for safety with oxygen therapy.

These safety precautions include education about the dangers of smoking and open flames, the avoidance of static electricity, avoiding the use of electric devices, such as electric razors near the oxygen therapy, keeping flammable materials, such as acetone, away from oxygen, keeping the oxygen canisters secure, and knowing the location of the nearest fire extinguisher.

Modifications of the Environment

Safe rooms and patient care areas are well lit and void of hazards. There should be no cords, wires, clutter, or other potential tripping hazards present. Rooms should be clean and dry, without risks of skidding or slipping. Rooms should have grab bars and handrails for patients, particularly in bathrooms and in areas where they walk. Chairs should be stable and equipped with armrests. Patient independence must be balanced with patient safety; thus, frequent monitoring is necessary.

Stabilization and Transport

Not all patients who come to the ER can be treated effectively and appropriately; nonetheless, all of these patients must be medically stabilized and then transported (by ambulance or helicopter) to a facility that has the capabilities to do so.

For example, many hospitals do not have the equipment, supplies and competent staff to care for multiple trauma patients or severe burn patients. These patients should be stabilized and transported to a trauma center or burn center.

Triage

Triage in the emergency department is the method by which patients are prioritized in terms of the urgency of their needs. The priorities are often established using Maslow's hierarchy of needs, with the ABCs as the greatest of all priorities. For example, a patient who has just appeared with chest pain takes priority over the child that has been waiting to be seen for a sore throat because this patient is at risk for the deterioration of the ABCs (airway, breathing, and cardiovascular functioning).

The Simple Triage and Rapid Treatment, or START model (or its abbreviated form) is often used for triage. START scores patients from zero (0) to 75 based on their severity.

Discharge Planning

Most patients return to the community after care in the emergency department. A good deal of patient and family education is done prior to discharge. Some aspects of this include teaching about pharmacological and non-pharmacological pain management strategies. When patients are discharged with pain medications, they must understand the use of the medication, the dosage, the frequency, side effects, interactions and adverse events that must be immediately reported to their doctor.

End of Life Issues

Organ and Tissue Donations

Organ and tissue donations, depending on the organ, can be donated by live donors or upon death. Most organs used for transplant are cadaver organs; others come from live donors who electively choose to donate. Emergency nurses must be aware of a patient's donor status when death is imminent so organs can be retrieved and transported to save the life of a person who needs a transplantation. There are no limitations in terms of the donor's age but organs are not donated when the person has cancer that is metastasizing, HIV/AIDS, severe infections and other conditions.

Some of the organs that can be donated for transplantation from a cadaver include the kidney, liver, pancreas, heart, lung and intestine. Live donors can donate whole kidneys and part of their liver, lung, intestine or pancreas. Tissues that can be donated for transplant are the skin, cornea, heart valves, bone, middle ear, veins, tendons, cartilage and ligaments. Some of the factors that are considered for deciding on an appropriate recipient include blood type, tissue type, the urgency of the recipient's health status, time spent on the waiting list and the geographic distance between the donor location and the recipient's geographic location.

The United Network for Organ Sharing (UNOS) maintains the Organ Procurement and Transplantation Network (OPTN), which matches donors and recipients 24 hours a day and 365 days a year recipients. Every transplant hospital is part of this network.

Advance Directives

Advance medical care directives (also known as living wills and advance directives) outline the patient's wishes regarding possible treatments available in case the patient is unable to competently consent to or reject treatment. For example, a person with no history of disease may elect to *not* have CPR or a ventilator in the event of sudden death. Another patient with cancer may choose to have tube feedings but no IVs in their advanced directive. The most commonly seen components of advance directives relate to life support measures, mechanical ventilation, administration of intravenous solution, and methods of artificial feeding, like tube feedings. Many patients at the end of life choose DNR (do not resuscitate), and they specifically state that they do not want mechanical ventilation, intravenous fluids and/or tube feedings. These directives should be as specific and complete as possible. When an unanticipated event or treatment occurs that is not included in these advance directives, decisions are made by the durable power of attorney for healthcare in the best interests of the patient and their values.

Family Presence at the End of Life

Death vigils vary among individuals, families, religions, cultures and ethnic groups. Individuals vary in terms of their physical and emotional attributes and strengths. Some choose to stay near their loved one at the end of their life, but others are unable. Some families prefer that only the nuclear family, rather than the extended family, stay close and support the loved one during their final hours and moments. Some religious practices include clergy to perform religious practices, such as the Catholics' Sacrament of the Sick; some cultures are welcoming of all loved ones and some have cultural practices and rituals for the end of life. Many ethnic groups have beliefs and practices regarding the end of life, including some relating to death vigil.

Nurses are a highly important part of the death vigil. They remain in presence, or readily available, to care for and support the dying patient and their loved ones. Simple measures such as providing privacy, a comfortable chair, coffee and meals are highly welcomed by family members. They also need the ongoing psychological and emotional support of the nurse at the end of life.

Some essential comfort and dignity measures that should be implemented at the end of life include the provision of comfort and privacy to loved ones and significant others as well as providing the patient with interventions that ensure clean, dry skin, clean bed linens, good oral hygiene and hydration with ice chips if possible. Other measures include proper turning and positioning, the management of incontinence, and the continuation of assessments and interventions like massage, pain management medications and treatment of any end of life symptoms.

The family members and/or loved ones of the patient, after death has occurred, are encouraged to acknowledge the pain of loss. The support and presence of the nurse allows the bereaved to express their feelings and to resolve their grief.

It is important that the bereaved not use any medications to suppress the pain of grieving. The nurse can support the family members and/or loved ones to grieve in a healthy, rather than a dysfunctional, manner. The acceptance of loss is the beginning phase of the healthy grieving process. Dysfunctional grieving is defined as an extended and unsuccessful resolution of grief. The nurse can facilitate healthy grieving by encouraging the loved ones to view, touch, hold and kiss the body of their loved one. The nurse can also provide emotional support after the death.

Withholding and Withdrawing Treatments

Nurses are required to withhold treatment when it is refused and documented without concerns about liability or negligence. There are also times when treatment can be legally and ethically withheld without refusal by the patient. For example, treatments can be legally withheld when they are deemed futile and when the patient is at the end of life due to a terminal disease or disorder. If it is unknown whether the disease is terminal and there is no patient refusal of treatment, such as an advance care directive, treatment must be rendered.

Palliative and Hospice Care

Hospice and palliative care nursing supports the patient by ensuring the best quality of life possible while relieving suffering up to the time of death. Hospice and palliative nursing also includes supporting the patient's family in the bereavement period. The ANA's Scope and Standards of Practice regarding Hospice and Palliative Nursing is the foremost authority in nursing on the subject. These standards of practice guide nurses providing end-of-life care. They also provide information on education, ethics and advocacy, communications, clinical judgment, and other professional issues. Finally, while the standards provide professional guidelines and support; however, laws regarding end-of-life care vary from state to state, affecting the hospice setting. In other words, the ANA's Scope and Standards of Practice is not a legal document.

The National Hospice and Palliative Care Organization (NHPCO) also provides extensive professional guidance on palliative and hospice care.

Pain Management

According to the International Association for the Study of Pain, pain management uses both pharmacological and non-pharmacological means to control a patient's pain; the goal of pain management is also to improve a patient's quality of life, enable work, recreation, and social engagement, and to allow for a dignified death.

Types of Pharmacological Pain Management Drugs

Opioids

An opioid is a natural or synthetic medication mediated by specific nervous system receptors. The most commonly used synthetic opioids are fentanyl and methadone; and some of the most commonly used natural opioids are morphine and codeine.

Drug	Range	Route	Indications
Codeine	30 mg q 4-6h	Oral	Mild to moderate pain
Fentanyl	50 mcg/hour (q 72h)	Oral, nasal, transdermal	Breakthrough pain
Hydrocodone	5-10 mg q 4-6h	Oral	Hydrocodone is available only in combination with other ingredients. Some hydrocodone products are used to relieve moderate to severe pain; other hydrocodone products are used to relieve cough.
Hydromorphone	2 mg 4-6h	Oral, injection, and rectal	Moderate to severe pain.
Methadone	2.5-5 mg BID-TID	Oral	Moderate to severe pain not relieved by non-narcotic pain relievers
Morphine	Immediate release 10 mg q 4h Sustained release 15 mg q 12h	Oral, rectal and injection	Moderate to severe pain

Oxycodone	Immediate release 5 mg q 4-6h Sustained release 10 mg q 12h	Oral	Moderate to severe pain
Oxymorphone	Immediate release 5-10 mg q 4-6h Sustained release 10 mg q 12h	Oral	Moderate to severe pain

Non-Opioids

A non-opioid is defined as a medication used for pain management that is not an opioid or considered an adjuvant.

Non-Steroidal Anti-Inflammatory Drugs (NSAIDS)

Drug	Range	Route	Indications
Naproxen	250-500 mg q 12h	Oral, rectal	Pain related to inflammatory conditions and chronic inflammatory conditions
Naproxen Na	275-550 mg q 12h	Oral	Pain and inflammation from muscular injuries
Oxaprozin	600-1200 mg q 24 h	Oral	Pain, stiffness and inflammation associated with rheumatoid and osteoarthritis
Aspirin	650-1000 mg q 4-6h	Oral	Pain, fever, and inflammation
Diflunisal	250-500 mg q 8-12h	Oral	Mild to moderate pain and inflammation
Salsalate	750-2000 mg q 12h	Oral	Pain, tenderness, swelling, and stiffness
Meclofenamate	50-100 mg q 6-8h	Oral	Mild to moderate pain, tenderness, swelling, and stiffness
Mefenamic acid	250 mg q 6h	Oral	Mild to moderate pain relief

Ketorolac (Toradol)	15-30 mg IV or IM q 6h or 20 followed by 10 mg q 4-6h	Oral, IM, IV and IV	Short-term management (up to 5 days) of moderately severe acute pain that otherwise would require narcotics
Diclofenac	50-100 mg, followed by 50 mg q 8h	Oral	Mild to moderate pain, fever and inflammation
Etodolac	200-400 mg q 6-8h	Oral	Inflammation and pain relief
Indomethacin	25-50 mg q 6-8h	Oral and rectal	Fever, pain and inflammation
Sulindac	150-200 mg q 12h	Oral	It is used for treating pain, fever, and inflammation.
Piroxicam	20-40 mg q 24h	Oral	Fever, pain, and inflammation
Acetaminophen	650-1000 mg q 6-8h	Oral	Acetaminophen relieves pain by elevating the pain threshold and it is also an antipyretic
Fenoprofen	200-600 mg q 6h	Oral	Mild to moderate pain, tenderness, swelling, and stiffness
Flurbiprofen	50-200 mg q 12h	Oral	Pain, tenderness, swelling, and stiffness relief
Ibuprofen	400mg q 4h to 800 mg q6h	Oral	Prescription strength and over the counter preparations are available. It relieves pain, tenderness, swelling, stiffness and fever
Ketoprofen	25-50 mg q 6-8h	Oral	Prescription strength and over the counter preparations are available. It is used to relieve pain, tenderness, swelling, stiffness, minor aches and pains from headaches, menstrual periods, toothaches, and backaches as well as an antipyretic
Celecoxib	100-200 mg q 12h	Oral	Pain, tenderness, swelling and stiffness

Anticonvulsants

Drug Name	Usual Dosage and Route	Indications for Pain Management
Carbamazepine	Oral dose two to four times a day Extended release tablet 2x/day	Chronic low back pain, cancer pain, and restless leg syndrome
Gabapentin	Oral once every 12 hours Extended release once a day	Chronic low back pain, cancer pain, and restless leg syndrome
Phenytoin	Oral two or three times a day Extended release capsules 1 to 3 times a day	Chronic low back pain, and cancer pain
Pregabalin	Oral capsule once daily	Chronic low back pain, cancer pain, and neuropathic pain
Topiramate	Oral twice a day (same time each day preferably morning and evening)	Chronic low back pain, cancer pain and prevention of migraine headaches
Carbamazepine	Oral two to four times a day and extended release tablet twice a day, and extended-release capsule twice a day	Cancer pain and facial nerve pain
Levetiracetam	Oral twice a day at the same time each day preferably in the morning and evening	Cancer pain
Oxcarbazepine	Oral twice a day at the same time each day preferably in the morning and evening	Cancer pain
Zonisamide	Oral capsule once or twice a day at the same time each day	Cancer pain
Valproic acid	Oral once a day	Restless leg syndrome

Tricyclic Antidepressants

Drug Name	Usual Dosage and Route	Indications for Pain Management
Amitriptyline	Oral one to four times a day	Neck pain, low back pain, chronic pelvic pain and chronic pain syndrome
Doxepin	Topical and oral capsule one to three times a day	Neck pain, low back pain, chronic pelvic pain, and chronic pain syndrome

Imipramine	Oral	Neck pain, low back pain, chronic pelvic pain, and chronic pain syndrome
Desipramine	Oral	Low back pain, and chronic pain syndrome
Nortriptyline	Oral	Low back pain, and chronic pain syndrome
Maprotiline	Oral	Low back pain
Trazodone	Oral	Chronic pelvic pain

Adjuvants

Adjuvant medications enhance the effects of opioids and non-opioids, treat symptoms that worsen pain (like anxiety), and provide pain relief for specific sources or sites.

Adjuvants include local anesthetics, anxiolytics and anticonvulsants. Topical local anesthetics are relatively new in pain management. Usually available over the counter, they act on pain by deadening the nerve endings in the skin. Invasive local anesthetics may also be used for severe pain. They include:

- *Peripheral nerve block* - local anesthetic is injected near a peripheral nerve to anesthetize that nerve's area of innervation.

- *Trans-incision (or Trans-wound) catheter anesthesia* - a multi-lumen catheter is inserted through an incision or wound to provide a local anesthetic.

- *Field block* – local anesthetic is injected subcutaneously into an area adjacent to the field to be anesthetized.

- *Plexus anesthesia* - local anesthetic is injected near a nerve plexus, generally inside a tissue compartment so that the drug is confined near the intended site of action. The anesthetic effect extends to the innervation areas of several or all nerves stemming from the plexus.

- *Epidural anesthesia* - a local anesthetic is injected into the epidural space and acts on the spinal nerve roots. The anesthetized area may include parts of the abdomen or chest or large regions of the body, depending on the injection site and amount of anesthesia used.

- *Intravenous regional anesthesia (Bier's block)* – a tourniquet is used to arrest the blood circulation of a limb; then local anesthetic is injected into a nearby vein, filling the limb's venous system and anesthetizing nerves and nerve endings throughout the tissues of the area deprived of blood circulation.

- *Infiltration anesthesia* - local anesthetic is injected directly into the tissue to be anesthetized.

- *Spinal anesthesia* - cerebrospinal fluid is injected with local anesthetic, usually at the lumbar spine (in the lower back). The anesthetic affects spinal nerve roots and part of the spinal cord, anesthetizing the area from the legs to the abdomen or chest.

Non-pharmacological Pain Interventions

The number and variety of non-pharmacological interventions including complementary, alternative and integrative modalities, are numerous and varied. Some patients prefer methods and modalities to others but there are many options; one or more may be highly beneficial for the patient.

Magnets

Although the benefits of magnets for pain have not been scientifically substantiated, according to the National Institutes of Health (NIH), and they can be associated with some undesired side effects, some people claim that they benefit from them. Some patients report relief of back pain, foot pain, arthritis pain and the pain associated with fibromyalgia.

Magnets, typically made of a metal like iron and alloys or mixtures of metals and/or non-metals, produce a magnetic field of different strengths as measured in terms of gauss. Magnets for pain relief typically have a strength of 300 to 5,000 gauss. To put this strength into context, these magnets are stronger than the magnetic field of the Earth and less than the magnets used for an MRI. Magnets may not be safe among patients with an insulin pump or pacemaker; they should be used alongside, not in lieu of, traditional and conventional pain relief measures.

Chiropractic Services

Many Americans seek chiropractic services, particularly when they are affected with acute or chronic back pain, headaches, and/or neck pain. Chiropractors use spinal manipulation and other treatments, including deep massage, to support the proper alignment of the body. It is believed that this manipulation restores mobility and decreases pain. Chiropractic care is usually considered safe but patients who have spinal cord compressions or who are taking anticoagulants should not use chiropractic spinal manipulation.

Homeopathy

Like other alternative treatments, homeopathic approaches to pain are not substantiated in literature and, despite the fact that homeopathic remedies are regulated by the FDA, this regulatory agency does not confirm their safety and effectiveness. Some of these remedies can also have adverse side effects.

Practitioners of homeopathic medicine believe that disorders and diseases can be treated with lower, highly diluted dosages rather than higher doses of a substance such as a plant, mineral or animal source. Some substances include low doses of mountain herb, red onions, white arsenic, stinging nettle and belladonna.

Massage

Massage decreases stress and pain. Relaxation techniques, soothing music and soft lighting combined with massage is a great way to help to alleviate stress and pain to promote sleep, rest and circulation. It also conveys caring and compassion as part of the nurse-patient relationship, and allows the nurse to communicate with the patient about their concerns. Massage can include hand massage, back massage, foot soaking and massage, and neck massage. A warm lotion or oil is used for massage.

Meditation

Meditation is thought to reduce fatigue, stress and anxiety. During meditation, the patient should be instructed to concentrate on one's breathing while repeating positive and calming phrases in one's mind. Meditation is spiritual, whereas prayer is often religious.

Prayer

These prayers can be formal or informal as well as religious and non-religious in nature.

Heat and Cold Applications

Heat and cold applications can be quite helpful in the reduction of pain. Heat can be helpful in reducing the pain associated with sore muscles. It can be applied with a heating pad, gel packet, warm water bottle or a hot bath or shower. Heat should not be used for more than ten minutes at a time.

Cold can help relieve or ease the pain in a patient by numbing it. Cold can be administered with cold gel packs, frozen peas or ice cubes wrapped in a cloth. Cold should be used for a maximum of ten minutes.

Deep Breathing

Deep breathing techniques are effective with tension, pain, anxiety and fatigue.

Progressive Muscular Relaxation

Progressive muscular relaxation (PMR) therapy aims to reduce tension, lower perceived stress, decrease pain and induce relaxation in the patient. It involves progressively tensing and releasing major skeletal muscle groups. Its goal is to reduce the stimulation of the autonomic and central nervous system and to increase parasympathetic activity.

It has been reported that patients who use progressive muscular relaxation experience a reduction in their state of anxiety, pain, symptoms of depression, and improve their sleeping habits as well as their overall quality of life.

Distraction

According to the American Cancer Society, distraction means turning your attention to something other than the pain. Distraction aims to manage mild pain and pain that occurs before an ordered analgesic medication takes effect. Some forms of distraction are watching television, talking on the telephone, or other things that can help the patient take their minds off of the pain they are experiencing.

Imagery

Imagery, which is also referred to as guided imagery or visualization, is mental exercises that are designed to allow the mind to influence the health and wellbeing of the body. The patient creates a kind of purposeful daydream by imaging sights, smells, tastes or other sensations.

Imagery is helpful in reducing stress, anxiety, depression, pain, and hypertension.

Biofeedback

Biofeedback is a method of treatment in which the patient is able to use monitoring devices to help consciously control physical processes that are normally controlled automatically. For example, temperature, heart rate, sweating, blood pressure, muscle tension and sweating can be controlled.

It has been shown that biofeedback can help patients with chronic pain, sleep difficulties and it can help to improve the patient's overall quality of life.

Hypnosis

Self-hypnosis and hypnosis produces a state that includes relaxation and deep concentration. It is helpful for reducing pain, fear, anxiety and fatigue among oncology patients.

Transcutaneous Nerve Stimulation (TENS)

A transcutaneous nerve stimulator, also referred to as a TENS unit, is used as a method of pain relief. TENS transmits low-voltage electrical impulses through electrodes placed on the skin on or around where the pain is. This nerve stimulation activates the body's pain modulatory pathways, thus decreasing the pain.

Acupuncture

This ancient Chinese medical treatment uses very thin needles, which are placed into the skin, and can help to reduce pain, nausea and vomiting.

Acupressure

Acupressure is similar to acupuncture, but it uses pressure instead of needless. It can be helpful in the treatment of anticipatory nausea.

Reiki

Reiki is another complementary healing approach. The therapist places their hands above the person, or lightly on the person, to facilitate the patient's own healing processes and responses.

This Eastern therapy is based on the belief that energy supports healing. A limited number of studies have indicate that there may be some benefits in terms of the symptoms of cancer, depression, pain, fibromyalgia, and depression.

Music Therapy

Music Therapy intends to enhance the patient's emotional, physical, cognitive and overall sense of wellbeing. Music therapists engage patients with singing, movement to music, creating music and listening to music. Many patients, particularly those who cannot speak, enjoy music as a form of alternative communication and stress reduction.

The four general types of music therapy are receptive, improvisation, recreative and creative. Receptive therapy includes things like listening to music and moving in rhythm or dancing; improvisation includes the active creation of music using voice sounds and musical instruments; recreative musical therapy includes recreational social activities like singing in a chorus; compositional music therapy includes creative songwriting and musical compositions.

Mind-Body Exercises

Mind-body exercises combine deep focused breathing, movement and meditation. These exercises can help the oncology patient combat stress, depression and fatigue. Yoga and tai chi are two examples of mind-body exercises.

Herbs

Herbs and dietary supplements are helpful for many oncology patients. Some herbs reduce vomiting and nausea; others help to decrease pain and fatigue. For example, astragalus, which comes from the astragalus plant's root, can boost the immune system. Vitamins like vitamins A, C, E and coenzyme Q 10 may provide some protection against cancer.

Many herbs and supplements are not documented in the literature as scientifically effective, and some can have side effects. It is necessary to instruct patients about the need to consult with their physician prior to the use of these substances.

System Concepts

Delegation to Assistive Personnel

Delegation is the transfer of the nurse's responsibility for the performance of a task to another nursing staff member while retaining accountability for the outcome. Responsibility can be delegated. Accountability *cannot* be delegated.

The "Five Rights of Delegation" are:

1. The "right" circumstances
2. The "right" person
3. The "right" task
4. The "right" directions and communication
5. The "right" supervision and evaluation

Proper delegation is crucial in nursing: ineffective and inappropriate delegation can lead to abysmal failures, the lack of goal achievement, illegal practice outside of the scope of practice, and jeopardy of the patient's safety. Delegating responsibilities for patient care to subordinates for whom those duties are beyond their scope of practice puts patients at risk and may even have life-threatening consequences.

In order to ensure high quality care, delegation must be appropriate. It follows that nurses must have an acute knowledge of the healthcare needs of patients; the abilities, competencies, job descriptions, and scope of practice of staff; the law; and policies and procedures.

Successful delegation balances the needs of the patients with abilities of attending staff in accordance with the law and established professional standards.

Those healthcare professionals delegating responsibilities to others must be well-informed about scopes of practice for each of their team members and the standards of care to be upheld. Delegated tasks must be aligned with the delegate's abilities according to the statutory scope of practice, standards of care and practice, and the facility's job description as well as policies and procedures related to the task.

When delegating care, nurses must consider the abilities and competencies of staff members. Each team member is different and unique. When possible, the personal preferences of the patient and the staff member should be accommodated for as long as the delegation is consistent with patient needs, the law, established policies, procedures, job descriptions and the competencies of the individual. The nurse must thoroughly and continuously supervise staff who have been delegated an aspect of care. The delegating nurse is fully accountable for all delegated tasks.

Disaster Management

Internal Disasters

Examples of internal disasters include fires, power losses, tornados, workplace violence, cyclones, hurricanes, and explosions. These situations are life endangering; there is little time to think and react.

Fires

Fires need heat, air, and something to burn. All three of these must be present for a fire to start, so eliminating one of these three ingredients is an important prevention method. Other flammables include solids like paper and wood, liquids like grease and gas such as fumes. Electricity is also flammable.

Fire prevention includes facility-wide smoke detectors and fire sprinklers, as well as established policies and procedures relating to smoking, oxygen use, electrical safety and the use of other gases like nitrous oxide. Facilities also need established policies and procedures to deal with fires and other internal and external disasters. All members of the facility must be fully knowledgeable about these procedures; when a disaster occurs there is no time to read the manual. Immediate action is necessary.

You *must* act quickly if a fire starts. You must R-A-C-E.

- **R -** Rescue everyone in danger; get all patients and visitors out of danger by following the fire plan set up by the facility you work in.

- **A -** Alarm; a fire alarm MUST be pulled.

- **C -** Confine or contain the fire. Close all doors and windows; fire doors are supposed to automatically close to contain a fire in a small area and to prevent its spread to other areas of the facility.

- **E -** Extinguish the fire, only if it is safe to do so and there is no possibility that you can injure yourself or anyone else. Small fires can be put out with water or a fire extinguisher when a solid is burning. If the fire is too large to handle, get out and wait for the professional firefighters or your facility's fire squadron.

When a fire occurs, you may be instructed to evacuate patients. The two methods of evacuation are vertical and horizontal. When you are instructed to do a vertical evacuation, you will move patients from one floor to another. For example, when a fire breaks out on the fourth floor, you will be instructed to move the patients to a lower level than the fourth floor because smoke and fire spreads upward. When you are instructed to horizontally evacuate patients, you will move them from one area of the floor to another area on the same floor as far away from the fire as possible.

All medical facilities must have emergency evacuation plans and they should be posted so that they can be referred to, and followed, in a rapid manner. Elevators are never used during a fire emergency. Elevators are reserved for firefighters and other emergency personnel, and elevators can lose electricity and trap people inside during a fire. The stairway is the only path of exit that can be used.

If a fire is blocking a patient's exit from their room, the door should be shut to keep the fire out of the room and a towel or blanket should be placed at the bottom of the door to keep the smoke out of their room. If a fire alarm sounds when you and/or your patient are in the room with the door closed, you must feel the door BEFORE opening it. A hot door means that the fire is just on the other side of the door so leave the door closed. Do *not* open it. Instead, put a towel or blanket at the bottom of the door to keep the smoke out and call for help.

Fire Extinguishers

Fire extinguishers are required at all medical facilities. There are several different types of fire extinguishers, which include:

- *Type A*: Type A fire extinguishers combat fires on paper, wood, cloth, and other solids. They are NOT suitable for oil, grease or electrical fires.

- *Type B*: Type B fire extinguishers combat gasoline, oil and grease fires; they can also put out kitchen fires (involving grease and fat). They are NOT suitable for electrical fires.

- *Type C*: Type C fire extinguishers combat electrical fires.

- Type *AB*: Type AB fire extinguishers combine type A and B fire extinguishers. They are suitable for use against fires on solids like paper, wood and cloth; they also combat gasoline, oil, grease, and kitchen fires (including grease and fat fires). They are NOT suitable for use on electrical fires.

- Type *BC*: Similar to type AB fire extinguishers, type BC fire extinguishers are a combination of the types B and C fire extinguishers. The type BC can be used on electrical, liquid and gas fires.

- Type *ABC*: Type ABC fire extinguishers are suitable for use against all fires; they should be present in all healthcare and medical facilities and homes. Type ABC fire extinguishers are available at most home improvement stores.

To ensure that they are ready for emergency use, fire extinguishers must be checked regularly. The P-A-S-S method provides a guide to the proper use of a fire extinguisher:

- Pull the pin
- Aim at the base, or the bottom, of the fire or flame
- Squeeze the trigger while holding the extinguisher up straight and
- Sweep, or move the spray, from side to side to completely cover the fire

What to do When a Patient's Clothes are on Fire

The rule for this disaster is to STOP, DROP AND ROLL. Tell the patient, or any other person, to STOP and DROP and NOT run. Running will add air to the fire. Fire victims should drop to the floor and shield their faces with their hands; roll them over repeatedly and cover them in a blanket to smother the flames. Do *not* fan a fire with your hands.

Smoke

If a room fills with smoke, the rule is to GET LOW AND GO. Smoke will fill a room from the ceiling down. Patients and visitors *must* get to the floor and crawl. As mentioned earlier, the door should be felt for heat and, if it is safe to exit, all persons present should cover their noses and mouths with wet rags and crawl out of danger.

Tornados and Serious Hurricanes

The following are steps that must be taken in case of a tornado:

- Go to the lowest level of the building near the center of a windowless interior room with no doors or walls adjacent to the outdoors. If you must take refuge in a room with windows, do NOT open them; close them quickly if you can. These measures protect people from flying debris.

- Close all interior doors in the building. If you are instructed to evacuate, do so.

- Keep curtains and blinds closed.

- Crouch or squat down low to the floor, and cover your face and head with your arms.

- If you are trapped under debris, cover your nose and mouth with a handkerchief or clothing to prevent dust from entering your airways.

Terrorism

Non-state actors use terrorism, or violence against civilians and non-military property and facilities, in order to effect political change. Terrorism may involve the use of chemical, biological, nuclear and radiological weapons, resulting in short- or long-term medical consequences and even death.

If an act of terrorism occurs in your facility, you *must* follow the instructions given to you by the facility because responses to these acts vary greatly in terms of the type of act and the severity. For example, you may be simply advised to be aware of your surroundings and to stay in place after a telephone bomb threat has been received.

External Disasters

Examples of external disasters include things like massive flooding, a nuclear explosion and a major train and school bus accident. The roles of nurses and other members of the organization vary, so it is highly important that you are very familiar with your organization's policies, procedures and protocols relating to all internal and external disasters. Emergency nurses, and all other members of the team, must respond rapidly to external disasters that bring large numbers of patients to healthcare facilities with varying needs and with little or no warning.

In most cases, victims of major disasters are transported from the field to the hospital after they have been triaged in the field. Color-coded tags are often used; these tags alert the emergency department staff to the severity of all arriving victims.

The four colors of triage:

Black	Expectant	Pain medication only until expected death
Red	Immediate	Life threatening injuries
Yellow	Delayed	Non-life threatening injuries
Green	Minimal	Minor injuries

Federal Regulations

The Health Insurance Portability and Accountability Act (HIPAA)

The Health Insurance Portability and Accountability Act (HIPAA) protects a patient's right to maintain the privacy and confidentiality of all his or her oral, written, and electronic medical information, unless the patient has provided express written consent to its disclosure. Access to all, or part, of the medical record is restricted to only those who have a "need to know". Many of those who have the "right to know and the need to know" are those who provide direct care to the patient; others who also have the legal "need to know" are those that provide indirect care and reimbursement. For example, a physical therapist, insurance companies, the case manager or a QA nurse may have a need to know even when they are not providing direct care to the patient because of the nature of their role.

Implications for the nurse in terms of HIPAA are numerous and the penalties for violations are severe. Some of the implications include prohibitions against discussing patients with others who do not have the "need to know", protecting patient's written records and logging off after accessing electronic medical records. Idle discussions about patients in the community, in the hospital elevator and/or cafeteria are prohibited; telephone conversations with unknown people without a code, or other unique identifier, are prohibited; logging off the computer and securing a hard copy chart so others cannot view them is mandatory; Facebook discussions and cell phone pictures are strictly prohibited.

Emergency Medical Treatment & Labor Act (EMTALA)

The Emergency Medical Treatment & Labor Act (EMTALA), passed in 1986, ensures that all people must have access to emergency care regardless of their ability to pay. Because of this federal law, all hospitals throughout the nation are mandated to provide stabilizing treatment for patients and/or stabilize and transport the patient.

Patient Rights

Informed Consent

Informed consents are legally and ethically necessary with few exceptions. Legally, informed consent prevents battery, assault and professional negligence. Ethically, informed consent upholds the ethical principles of self-determination and patient autonomy. Consent can be written, oral and implied. Written consents are the best of all types; however, there are times when oral and implied consent is necessary. For example, a patient in an ER may be competent and capable of giving an oral consent to treatment until they are stable enough to provide a written consent.

Implied consent is defined as consent to assessments or treatments by the nature of the consent for hospitalization or treatment. There are four elements of a valid, legal, ethical and complete consent. Consent is given freely without any undue coercion or influence, the patient has the cognitive capacity to give consent or refuse a treatment, the consent is specific in terms of the procedure or treatment, and the patient fully comprehends the information given to them about the treatment or procedure, its benefits, its risks and alternatives.

Emergency lifesaving treatment can be carried out without consent when the treatment is urgent and necessary to preserve health and wellbeing. Minor treatments can also be done without consent when the person (parent or guardian) cannot be contacted.

The Patients' Bill of Rights and Patient Responsibilities

According to the American Hospital Association, all patients have the right to:

- Respect and dignity
- Choose their own doctor(s)
- Privacy
- Confidentiality
- Freedom from abuse and neglect
- Control their finances and personal property
- Know about their medical condition and treatments
- Make decisions about their medical care
- Competent care
- Religious and social freedom
- Accurate bills for services given
- Complain and be heard

Patients also have responsibilities relating to their behavior and medical care. They are responsible to give complete information relating to their past and present health concerns and conditions, including medications, signs and symptoms. They must communicate safety concerns and any lack of understanding relating to their state of health and treatments, or interventions.

Patients are also responsible for actively participating in all aspects of care and treatment, including discharge planning, and providing accurate and current health insurance information. Patient behavior responsibilities include following all the facility's policies and procedures and acting in a manner that is cooperative as well as considerate of the rights of others.

Performance Improvement

Measuring quality has evolved over the years from quality control, to quality assurance, quality improvement to performance improvement and continuous quality improvement. It has also evolved from structure studies to process studies to outcome-related studies. Successful quality management and performance improvement activities improve the outcomes of care; they improve the safety and efficiency of processes, and reduce costs, risks and liability.

These activities are mandated by external regulatory bodies such as the Joint Commission on the Accreditation of Healthcare Organizations (JCAHO), the Centers for Medicare and Medicaid (CMS) and state departments of health. Quality management is an integral part of the nurse's role and every healthcare provider's responsibility. Efforts should focus on areas with the greatest risk, the greatest volume, the highest costs and the most problem prone.

Although models differ somewhat, continuous quality or performance improvement activities include the identification of an opportunity to improve a process, organizing a team to work on the improvement activity *which includes those closely related to the process) identifying patient expectations and outcomes, gathering data and information, including best practices and research studies, and analyzing the data. It also includes the close examination of existing processes, designing processes with measurable specifications that can be evaluated, the elimination of all variances, the implementation of newly designed processes, the evaluation of improvement or innovation in terms of measurable specifications, and the documentation of the entire process that led to the change or improvement.

Quality indicators can be categorized as core measures and outcome measures. Core measures are standardized measures of quality. The Joint Commission on the Accreditation of Healthcare Organizations (JCAHO) has ORYX National Hospital Quality Measures that include disease-related measures, such as heart failure and pneumonia, population measures, such as pediatric care, and organizational measures, like those used in intensive care areas.

Outcome measures are used to examine the outcomes of care. For example, mortality and morbidity rates, infection rates after surgery, MRSA rates, patient satisfaction findings, lengths of stay and readmissions may be analyzed as an outcome measure.

Structure, processes and outcomes can be evaluated with quantitative or qualitative data. The prevalence or incidence of falls and nosocomial infections are examples of quantitative data. Patient satisfaction and quality of life are often anecdotal narrative comments. This is considered qualitative data although these two anecdotal levels can also be quantified using a quantitative measurement scale or tool so they can be analyzed and evaluated with statistical analysis.

Outcomes will be unpredictable and filled with variances if the process and the structure are not stable. Unstable structures and processes will lead to unstable outcomes. The goal is to achieve and maintain stable and predictable high-quality outcomes, so good structures and processes must be in place and concretized before outcomes can be stabilized, improved and optimized.

Nurses can, and should, measure outcomes relating to physiological or biological health problems, psychological status, quality of life, functional abilities, the prevention of infections, goal attainment, safety, and the occurrence of adverse events. This can involve the measurement of performance over time in a longitudinal manner to determine if planned changes have sustained increased performance, and to identify problems and opportunities for improvement.

Peer Review

Professional peers can collaborate to identify opportunities for improvement and work together to critically evaluate aspects of care.

Variance Tracking

There are four types of variance including practitioner variance, system/institutional variance, community variance and patient/family variances. In the context of continuous quality improvement, a variance is a quality defect. Variances can be random or specific. A random variance is one that occurs because of things inherent to the process; these variances occur each time the established process is carried out. Specific variances occur because of one specific part of the process. Both of these variances indicate that efforts must be made to correct and eliminate variance.

Benchmarking and Best Practices

Benchmarking and the identification of best practices are superior ways to objectively determine quality and risk. Some hospitals provide care that is less costly, some hospitals achieve better patient outcomes and some hospitals have lower incidences of sentinel events than others do. Nurses should identify these best practices and attempt to replicate them to continuously improve quality.

Data Management

Data can be collected and analyzed to measure individual and group outcomes. For example, a emergency department nurse may use data to measure the effectiveness of a program, like infection control, or the outcomes of care for aggregated populations, such as the outcomes of care for a population of patients who are affected with a specific ailment.

Risk Management

Risk management is closely aligned with continuous quality improvement, but instead of proactively planning change like quality improvement, risk management aims to reduce liability by eliminating risks and liabilities. These can include patient-related risks, quality risks and financial risks and liabilities.

Risk management identifies and eliminates hazards relating to basic safety such as falls, elopement, infant abduction, a wide variety of medical errors such as wrong site surgery, wrong patient surgery and medication errors. JCAHO has requirements relating to medical errors in terms of reporting sentinel events and the elimination of hazards using root cause analysis.

The main concepts behind risk management include the identification of any potential risks that can occur, analyzing the likelihood of a risk occurring, what effects the risk can have, the cost associated with the risk, and consideration of how the risk can be controlled and, if possible, eliminated. Prevention of all negative outcomes, which could potentially lead to a lawsuit or claim, is necessary.

Nurses must identify patients who are vulnerable to high-risk incidents. For example, all patients should be screened for falls risk, infection risk, and skin breakdown. Immediate and specific preventive measures are put in place for all "at risk" patients.

In order to avoid making mistakes, the institution should have clear policies, efficient working practices, well-defined responsibilities, adequate communication and sufficient staff assigned to work according to their documented and validated level of competency. In addition to patient-related risks, environmental risks like faulty equipment, hazardous materials, hazardous waste, fire and security issues place patients, staff and visitors at risk.

Root Cause Analysis

Root cause analysis is a process used to dig down to the real reasons why mistakes and errors have occurred. These reasons are usually procedures and processes, *not* people. Root cause analysis occurs in a blame-free environment with teams of stakeholders who closely analyze faulty processes with a number of techniques such as brainstorming, flow charting, fishbone diagrams, data collection and statistical data analysis.

It is recommended that all sentinel events are examined using root cause analysis. A sentinel event is an occurrence that leads to, or has the potential to lead to, an adverse outcome. For example, when a patient has a left leg amputation instead of a right leg amputation, it leads to liability and actual harm. On the other hand, when a nurse is about to administer an incorrect medication or dosage and they suddenly realize that they are about to err and they stop and correct the dosage it is also a sentinel event. Even "near misses" are considered sentinel events.

The processes that cause harm as well as those that lead to "near misses" must be refined and improved so that all possible human errors are eliminated and future sentinel events can be prevented.

Some of the most commonly occurring medical error sentinel events include the unintended retention of a foreign body after surgery or another invasive procedure, wrong patient/wrong site/ wrong procedure, treatment delays, suicide, operative and post-operative complications, falls, criminal events, medication errors, perinatal death and other unanticipated events.

Practice Examination

1. Which of the following statements about abdominal aneurysms is true?
   A. Most are asymptomatic.
   B. Cerebral arteries are affected.
   C. They are associated with atherosclerosis.
   D. They most often lead to immediate death.

2. Automatic electronic defibrillators are intended for use by:
   A. EMTs in the community.
   B. ACLS certified nurses.
   C. BLS and ACLS certified nurses.
   D. All people in the community.

3. Select the cardiac arrhythmia that is accurately paired with its etiology or cause.
   A. Paroxysmal supraventricular tachycardia: The AV junction takes over the SA node function.
   B. Atrial flutter: Occurs when there are cyclical vagal variations in the sinus rhythm.
   C. Sinus arrhythmia: Results when the AV node blocks rapid atrial depolarization rates of about 300 beats per minute.
   D. Atrial fibrillation: Occurs when the SA node depolarizes quicker than normal.

4. Which patient is at greatest risk for endocarditis?
   A. An artificial heart recipient
   B. All organ transplant recipients
   C. Males less than 30 years of age
   D. Males over 30 years of age

5. **Which disorder is characterized with Osler's nodes?**
   A. Rheumatoid arthritis
   B. Bacterial arthritis
   C. Temporal arteritis
   D. Endocarditis

6. **Select the type of heart failure that is accurately paired with one of its risk factors.**
   A. Left ventricular failure: Systemic hypertension
   B. Right ventricular failure: Anemia
   C. Right ventricular failure: Myocardial infarction
   D. Biventricular heart failure: Aortic stenosis

7. **The goal of treatment for hypertensive crisis is to decrease the blood pressure by about:**
   A. 20% in 1hour.
   B. 30% in 1hour.
   C. 20% in ½ hour.
   D. 30% in ½ hour.

8. **Which patient is at greatest risk for deep vein thrombosis?**
   A. An adult who has travelled to NY with a 10 hour train trip
   B. An adult who has travelled to NY with a 4 hour plane trip
   C. An active child who has travelled to NY with a 10 hour train trip
   D. An active child who has travelled to NY with a 4 hour plane trip

9. **A vena cava filter is often used for the treatment of which serious and life threatening disorder?**
   A. Cardiac tamponade
   B. Deep vein thrombosis
   C. Pneumothorax
   D. Hemothorax

10. Which patient is at greatest risk for cardiac tamponade?
    A. A 67 year old male with a pneumothorax
    B. A 67 year old male with a hemothorax
    C. A patient with hypovolemic shock
    D. A patient with obstructive shock

11. A 17 year old male presents with severe pain in the lower right quadrant of the abdomen and complaints of nausea and projectile vomiting. The muscles in his abdomen are rigid and he reports that pulling his knees up relieves the pain somewhat. His fever is 100.7 degrees Fahrenheit; his white cell count is 15,000/mm3, and neutrophils of 80%. What is he most likely suffering from?
    A. Appendicitis
    B. Upper GI obstruction
    C. Cholecystitis
    D. Cholithiasis

12. In what part of the gastrointestinal tract do Mallory Weiss tears occur?
    A. Stomach
    B. Esophagus
    C. Small intestine
    D. Large intestine

13. Which statement about cholecystitis and/or cholelithiasis is accurate?
    A. Hypercholesterolemia is a risk factor associated with cholelithiasis
    B. African Americans are at greater risk for both when compared to Caucasians
    C. Cholecystitis is the formation of primarily calcium gall stones
    D. Acalculous cholecystitis usually occurs after a serious burn

14. What gastrointestinal disorder is characterized with a positive Murphy's sign?
    A. Appendicitis
    B. Cholecystitis
    C. Septic bowel
    D. Malabsorption

15. Which circulatory problem can develop when hepatic scar tissue blocks the normal flow of blood?
    A. Portal hypertension
    B. Portal hypotension
    C. Esophageal varices
    D. Aortic aneurysm

16. Which gastrointestinal disorder can result from the abnormal flow of blood to the liver?
    A. Esophageal atresia
    B. Esophageal varices
    C. Malabsorption
    D. Diverticulitis

17. Barrett's esophagus is a serious complication of which disorder?
    A. Endocarditis
    B. Esophagitis
    C. Liver cirrhosis
    D. Gastric acid reflux disease

18. A surgical treatment of esophageal varices is:
    A. A transjugular intrahepatic portosystemic shunt (TIPS)
    B. A transcutaneous intrahepatic portosystemic shunt (TIPS)
    C. A temporary intrahepatic portosystemic shunt (TIPS)
    D. A transmittive intrahepatic portosystemic shunt (TIPS)

19. A six year old child presents at the emergency room after accidently drinking ammonia. He is experiencing heartburn, melena, diarrhea, nausea and vomiting, and epigastric pain. Antacids are able to provide some relief. His temperature is 101 degrees Fahrenheit. What is the most likely diagnosis?
    A. Acute gastritis
    B. Chronic gastritis
    C. Esophagitis
    D. Gastroenteritis

20. **Which age group is most at risk for the complications of gastroenteritis?**
    A. A preschool child
    B. A school age child
    C. A neonate
    D. An adolescent

21. **What are the phases of hepatitis in correct sequential order?**
    A. The induction phase, the pre-icteric phase, the icteric phase and the post-icteric phase
    B. The pre-icteric phase, the induction phase, the icteric phase and the post-icteric phase
    C. The pre-icteric phase, the post-icteric phase and the icteric phase
    D. The pre-icteric phase, the icteric phase and the post-icteric phase

22. **Dark urine and clay colored stool are an indication of:**
    A. Dehydration
    B. Cholecystitis
    C. Hepatitis
    D. Portal hypertension

23. **During which phase of hepatitis does jaundice and pruritus occur?**
    A. Induction phase
    B. Post-icteric phase
    C. Pre-icteric phase
    D. Icteric phase

24. **Exposures to hepatitis A and B are prophylactically treated with a(n):**

    A. Passive, artificial immunity agent
    B. Active, artificial immunity agent
    C. Natural, active immunity agent
    D. Natural, passive immunity agent

25. **What is the most common type of hernia?**
    A. Inguinal
    B. Hiatal
    C. Umbilical
    D. Incisional

26. **Select the statement that is accurate and true relating to Crohn's Disease.**
    A. The typical area of intestinal involvement is the left colon and rectum.
    B. The extent of involvement usually is diffuse throughout the entire small intestine.
    C. The extent of involvement is noncontagious and segmented.
    D. The inflammation is mostly mucosal and bacterial in nature.

27. **Which age group is at greatest risk for intussusception?**
    A. The elderly because they most often have dysphagia
    B. The elderly because of the normal changes of the aging process
    C. Children because they most often swallow foreign bodies
    D. Children because of a gastrointestinal abnormality

28. **What is the initial treatment of pancreatitis focused on?**
    A. Reducing the inflammation of the pancreas
    B. A cholecystectomy
    C. Draining the fluid from the pancreas
    D. Removal of the bile duct obstruction

29. **What type of ulcer should the nurse be most aware of after a patient has suffered from a massive burn injury?**
    A. Gastric ulcers
    B. Cushing's ulcer
    C. Peptic ulcers
    D. Curling's ulcer

30. **Which fact about urinary tract infections is accurate?**
    A. Males are at greater risk for urinary tract infections than females.
    B. Females are at less risk for urinary tract infections than males.
    C. Klebsiella is the most common pathogen associated with urinary tract infections
    D. Indwelling urinary catheters place patients at risk for urinary tract infections

31. **What virus is orchitis most commonly associated with?**
    A. Measles
    B. Mumps
    C. Malaria
    D. Chicken pox

32. **When the spermatic cord that supports the testes in the scrotum is twisted, it is referred to as:**
    A. Testicular torsion.
    B. Priapism.
    C. Phimosis.
    D. An inguinal hernia.

33. **Urinary retention is defined as:**
    A. 35% or more of residual after voiding.
    B. 45% or more of residual after voiding.
    C. More than 100 ml of residual after voiding.
    D. More than 200 ml of residual after voiding.

34. **A 25 year old woman presents at the emergency room complaining of a painful, tender lump near her vaginal opening. She informs the staff that it is causing discomfort when she sits down, walks and has intercourse. Her temperature is 101.5 degrees Fahrenheit. What is the most likely diagnosis for this patient?**
    A. She has a Bartholin's cyst
    B. She has toxic shock syndrome
    C. An ectopic pregnancy
    D. She has pelvic inflammatory disease

35. Dysmenorrhagia is:

  A. Vaginal bleeding that occurs at a time other than during the normal menstrual cycle.

  B. Irregular and/or heavy vaginal bleeding that occurs without a known cause.

  C. Marked with cramping and pain during menstruation.

  D. Often associated with metrorrhagia, menorrhagia, and post-coital bleeding.

36. Select the condition that is correctly matched with its etiology.

  A. Tubo-ovarian abscess: Caused by staphylococcus aureus and streptococcal pathogens

  B. Endometritis: An inflammation or infection of the vas deferens

  C. Salpingitis: An inflammation or infection of the fallopian tubes

  D. Toxic shock syndrome: Caused by pelvic inflammatory disease, acute salpingitis, or post miscarriage

37. Select the term correctly matched with the statement.

  A. Battery: The threat of harm or a perceived threat

  B. Battery: Actual touching of a person without their consent regardless of whether or not harm was done

  C. Assault: Actual touching of a person without their consent regardless of whether or not harm was done

  D. Assault: Can only occur with physical contact

38. A 32 year old woman presents in the emergency department complaining of severe nausea and vomiting, weight loss, lightheadedness, and fainting. She informs the personnel that she just found out she is six weeks pregnant. What is the most likely diagnosis?

  A. Ectopic pregnancy

  B. Hyperemesis gravidarum

  C. Threatened abortion

  D. Preeclampsia

39. What percentage of neonates require some degree of neonatal resuscitation at delivery?
    A. 5%
    B. 10%
    C. 15%
    D. 20%

40. What is the ultimate cure for preeclampsia, eclampsia, and HELLP syndrome?
    A. Blood pressure management
    B. Magnesium sulfate
    C. Delivery of the baby
    D. Treating active seizures as they occur

41. Preterm labor occurs when contractions occur and the cervix begins to dilate prior to:
    A. 30 weeks of pregnancy.
    B. 35 weeks of pregnancy.
    C. 37 weeks of pregnancy.
    D. 40 weeks of pregnancy.

42. Treatment for a peritonsillar abscess includes:
    A. Vaginal irrigation.
    B. NSAIDS.
    C. Antibiotics and pus drainage.
    D. Salt water rinses.

43. A patient presents with epistaxis, what position should they be told to stay in?
    A. Lying back with the head even with the body
    B. Lying back with the head back
    C. Upright and with the head forward
    D. Upright and with the head backward

44. An eight year-old child presents in the emergency department complaining of a sore throat, pain, headache, malaise, ear discharge and tugging at their ear lobe. Upon examination swelling and redness are seen over the bone interior to the pinna, as well as a lumpy, yellowish tympanic membrane. The patient's fever is 101.3 degrees Fahrenheit. The child's mother informs the personnel that the patient just got over an upper respiratory infection. What is the most likely diagnosis?

    A. Acute otitis media
    B. Otitis externa
    C. Mastoiditis
    D. Labyrinthitis

45. A 38 year old female comes to the ER complaining that, over the last few days, she has been experiencing vertigo, nausea, vomiting, loss of balance, tinnitus, hearing loss, and a rushing noise in the ear. She informs the nurse that the symptoms become more intense when she moves her head, sits up, looks upward, and rolls over. Initial testing indicates that she has no neurological deficits. What is the most likely diagnosis?

    A. Otitis media
    B. Acute otitis media
    C. Labyrinthitis
    D. Meniere's disease

46. A 45 year-old male comes to the ER complaining of vertigo, nausea and vomiting, hearing loss, tinnitus, and a feeling of increased pressure in the ear. He notifies the personnel that he had a similar episode a few months before, but that it only lasted for five hours, and this episode has been occurring for six hours already. What is the most likely diagnosis?

    A. Otitis media
    B. Acute otitis media
    C. Labyrinthitis
    D. Meniere's disease

47. **Select the statement that describes the treatment or symptoms of a corneal abrasion.**
    A. Patients must stop contact lens use for at least two to three days
    B. Antibiotic treatment is necessary to cure and control it.
    C. Symptoms include clouding of the cornea and cornea melting.
    D. Peripheral vision deteriorates slowly over time.

48. **Which symptom or treatment is most likely when a patient presents with an ocular chemical burn?**
    A. Antibiotics are never be used for treatments.
    B. Symptoms include clouding of the cornea and corneal melting.
    C. Symptoms include clouding of the iris and corneal melting.
    D. Normal saline irrigations are avoided.

49. **Select the type of glaucoma that is accurately paired with its description.**
    A. Primary open-angle glaucoma: Peripheral vision remains clear
    B. Primary open-angle glaucoma: A medical emergency that must be treated immediately
    C. Acute angle-closure glaucoma: Gradual loss of peripheral vision
    D. Acute angle-closure glaucoma: A medical emergency that must be treated immediately

50. **Anterior uveitis is another term for:**
    A. Conjunctivitis
    B. Iritis
    C. Hyphema
    D. Nasolacrimal tearing

51. **Bleeding between the cornea and iris is referred to as:**
    A. Retinal artery occlusion
    B. Retinal detachment
    C. Hyphema
    D. Nasolacrimal tearing

52. **Your ER patient has presented with hyphema. The ophthalmologist has assessed the patient and determined that the blood level is more than 1/3 but less than 2/3. What grade hyphema does this patient have?**
   A. Grade one
   B. Grade two
   C. Grade three
   D. Grade four

53. **Which is the greatest treatment priority for a patient with a globe rupture?**
   A. Emergency fluid replacement to maintain ocular moisture
   B. Eye drops to prevent the expulsion of intraocular contents
   C. Immediate placement in a flat position
   D. Aggressive pain management to prevent the expulsion of intraocular contents

54. **Your patient has noninfectious keratitis as a result of wearing contact lenses for an extended period of time. She is being discharged into the community. What should you teach her about?**
   A. The need for a patch for at least 24 hours
   B. The need for antifungal eye drops for 5 days
   C. The need for lying flat for at least 24 hours
   D. The dangers of using a computer

55. **A major difference between delirium and dementia is that delirium is:**
   A. Persists for less than 3 days and dementia lasts longer.
   B. Is typically progressive until unconsciousness occurs.
   C. Sometimes reversible and dementia is not.
   D. Barely detectable and dementia is obvious.

56. **What medications are used to treat myasthenia gravis?**
   A. Anticholinesterases, such as pyridostigmine
   B. Opioid analgesics such as codeine and fentanyl
   C. Anticonvulsants such as carbamazepine
   D. Tricyclic antidepressants such as doxepin

57. **Normal intracranial pressure ranges from:**
     A. 3 to 10 mmHg.
     B. 5 to 15 mmHg.
     C. 8 to 17 mmHg.
     D. 10 to 20 mmHg.

58. **Which of the following statements about meningitis is accurate?**
     A. Bacterial meningitis is the most common form of meningitis.
     B. Significant mortality and morbidity are associated with viral meningitis.
     C. Bacterial meningitis symptoms mimic those of systematic infection.
     D. The meningitis vaccine has serious side effects among children, including autism.

59. **Your pediatric patient's mother reports to you that her child has been having seizures that last only about 10 seconds while she is sleeping. What education should you provide this mother with?**
     A. Information about tonic seizures
     B. The treatment of tonic-clonic seizures
     C. The prevention of myoclonic seizures
     D. The signs and symptoms of atonic seizures

60. **Which patient is at greatest risk for spinal cord compression?**
     A. A 26 year old male patient with lymphoma
     B. A 56 year old post menopausal woman
     C. An 86 year old male with primary cancer of the testes
     D. A 35 year old with disseminated intravascular coagulation

61. **Which statement about ischemic stroke is accurate?**
     A. 15% of patients with acute ischemic stroke have seizures
     B. Anticoagulants are recommended for patients with acute ischemic stroke
     C. Immediate administration of aspirin can reduce mortality and recurrent stroke
     D. Aspirin is not recommended for ischemic stroke patients

62. **Select the type of amputation that is accurately paired with its description.**
    A. Closed amputation: Used when the limb is infected
    B. Closed amputation: The muscle and bone are cut at the same level
    C. Opened amputation: The most common type of amputation used for diabetic patients
    D. Traumatic amputation: Results from pressure and fragmentation of bone

63. **Which patient is at greatest risk for compartment syndrome?**
    A. A 76 year old paraplegic patient with disuse syndrome
    B. A post menopausal woman with low bone density
    C. A healthy 6 year old who broke his leg
    D. A person who has second degree burns

64. **A 56 year-old woman comes to the ER complaining of chronic pain and tenderness on the left side of her breastbone. She explains that the pain is felt on several ribs and gets worse when she breaths deeply and when she coughs. What is the most likely diagnosis?**
    A. Tietze syndrome
    B. A sternal fracture
    C. Osteomyelitis
    D. Compartment syndrome

65. **Select the type of fracture correctly paired with its description.**
    A. Stable fracture: Likely to be displaced so it requires reduction
    B. Open fracture: A simple fracture of the lower extremity
    C. Incomplete fracture: Only one part of the bone is affected
    D. Pathological fracture: A compound fracture that breaks through the skin

66. **Select the correctly paired Garden classification for femoral neck fractures and its description.**
    A. Grade I: Displaced
    B. Grade II: Nondisplaced
    C. Grade III: completely displaced
    D. Grade IV incompletely displaced

67. What is the most common cause of osteomyelitis?

    A. Streptococcus

    B. Staphylococcus

    C. Escherichia coli

    D. Epstein Barr

68. What physical force places a patient at risk for pressure ulcers?

    A. Poor nutrition

    B. Immobility

    C. Shearing

    D. Gravity

69. Which musculoskeletal complication of immobility is common?

    A. Skeletal remineralization

    B. Contractures

    C. Super pronation

    D. Muscular extension

70. You have delegated some aspects of care to the nursing assistant. He is caring for several immobile patients who are on bed rest. How often should this nursing assistant minimally run and reposition these immobile patients?

    A. Every 15 minutes

    B. Twice an hour

    C. Every hour

    D. Every 2 hours

71. A 6 year-old child presents in the emergency department after stepping on a rusty nail. Upon examination, you notice that it is a deep wound that is not bleeding very much. What type of injury would you suspect?

    A. A serious abrasion

    B. A serious laceration

    C. A puncture wound

    D. An impact injury

72. Your patient presents with an avulsion in which a part of the skin on their hand is completely torn off from the underlying tissue. What type of injury is this classified as?
    A. A puncture wound
    B. A de-gloving injury
    C. An abrasion
    D. A laceration

73. A man threatens to isolate his family and not allow the family members to leave the house for any reason if they continue to "spend his money". This is an example of:
    A. Physical neglect
    B. Physical abuse
    C. Psychological abuse
    D. Financial neglect

74. A patient comes to the ER complaining of increased helplessness, irritability, insomnia, vigilance, fright and worry. What types of psychological symptoms of anxiety are they experiencing?
    A. Affective and behavioral symptoms
    B. Psychological and cognitive symptoms
    C. Parasympathetic and affective symptoms
    D. Cognitive and parasympathetic symptoms

75. A 35 year-old woman presents to the emergency room with hyperventilation, tachycardia, dizziness, and shortness of breath. You note that she is speaking in a rapid speed and seems to be confused. What level of anxiety is she experiencing?
    A. Mild
    B. Moderate
    C. Severe
    D. Panic level

76. Your patient has terminal cancer and the patient's daughter has expressed extreme sorrow about their mother and their mother's impending death. What type of loss is this daughter most likely experiencing?
    A. Perceived loss
    B. Anticipatory loss
    C. Actual loss
    D. Profound loss

77. Which theorist has shock, awareness of the loss, conservation, healing and renewal as the phases of bereavement?
    A. Sander
    B. Kubler-Ross
    C. Engel
    D. Piaget

78. The first three phases of grieving in correct sequential order, according to Engel's theory, include:
    A. Shock and disbelief, developing awareness and restitution.
    B. Developing awareness, shock and renewal.
    C. Developing awareness, shock and restitution.
    D. Shock, awareness of the loss and conservation and withdrawal.

79. Whose theory of grieving includes the unique phase of bargaining?
    A. Engel's
    B. Sander's
    C. Maslow's
    D. Kubler Ross's

80. Under what circumstance can confidentiality be legally violated?
    A. When the patient is infected with a terminal disease
    B. When the patient expresses thoughts of suicide
    C. When the patient is unable to speak
    D. When the patient is unable to see

81. **What are the most common causes of a malignant pleural effusion?**
    A. Lung and breast cancer
    B. Colon and prostate cancer
    C. Stomach and kidney cancer
    D. Ovarian and colon cancer

82. **Select the disorder that is correctly paired with its description.**
    A. Pneumothorax: Occurs when blood leaks into the area between the chest wall and lungs
    B. Pneumothorax: Occurs when clear fluid leaks into the area between the chest wall and lungs
    C. Hemothorax: Occurs when blood leaks into the area between the chest wall and lungs
    D. Hemothorax: Occurs when clear fluid leaks into the area between the chest wall and lungs

83. **A patient comes to the ER with hypoxia, tachypnea, and hypotension. The patient has suffered a laceration of their left lung and their trachea. You assess that the mediastinum has shifted to the right side. What is the most likely diagnosis?**
    A. Tension pneumothorax
    B. Pulmonary embolus
    C. Ruptured aortic aneurysm
    D. Hemothorax

84. **A four year-old boy presents with a burn that affects 8% of the total body surface. What type of burn does he have?**
    A. A minor burn
    B. A third-degree burn
    C. A moderate level burn
    D. A severe burn

85. **A patient presents with a viper snake bite. What is the antivenom of choice?**
    A. Taipan antivenom
    B. Vipera tab
    C. Viper tab antivenom
    D. Death adder antivenom

86. **What types of poisonous snakes are indigenous to the United States?**
    A. Rattlesnakes, death adder, and pseudechis spp.
    B. Rattlesnakes, copperhead snakes, and taipan
    C. Rattlesnakes, death adder, and taipan
    D. Rattlesnakes, copperhead snakes, and coral snakes

87. **Select the stage of shock that is accurately paired with its symptoms.**
    A. Initial Stage: Lactic acid builds up
    B. Compensatory Stage: Blood pH decreases
    C. Progressive Stage: Respiratory acidosis worsens
    D. Refractory Stage: Compensatory mechanisms begin

88. **Your patient is suffering from listeria poisoning. What treatment would you anticipate rendering to this patient?**
    A. Activated charcoal
    B. Gastric lavage
    C. Oral antibiotics as soon as possible
    D. IV antibiotics as soon as possible

89. **Which parasite is primarily found in regions and areas with poor sanitation and unsafe water?**
    A. Ring worm
    B. Tineas
    C. Scabies
    D. Giardia

90. **An eight year-old boy comes to the ER with a large dry, cracked, red, rash that looks like a burn on his left shin up to his knee. His mother informs you that she noticed it the night before after the boy was playing hide and seek with friends in the wooded backyard. He has been complaining of severe itchiness. What is the most likely diagnosis?**
    A. Poison ivy poisoning
    B. Lyme's disease
    C. Ringworm
    D. Brown recluse spider bite

91. **An 18 month-old child comes to the ER with her mother. Her mother states that she found her little girl drinking toilet bowl cleaner. You are not sure about what chemicals or toxins are in toilet bowl cleaners so you call the Poison Control Center. What will the Poison Control Center tell you about toilet bowl cleaners and/or the child's emergency treatment?**
    A. "Toilet bowl cleaners contain aspergillus fumigates so induce immediate vomiting"
    B. "Toilet bowl cleaners increase carbon monoxide levels so bring the child outdoors immediately"
    C. "Toilet bowl cleaners contain sulfuric acid so provide for immediate respiratory support"
    D. "Toilet bowl cleaners contain sulfuric acid so immediately induce vomiting"

92. **A couple comes to the ER by ambulance. EMS informs you that they observed dinner cooking on a barbecue in the kitchen and the couple was losing consciousness. What are they most likely suffering from?**
    A. Carbon monoxide poisoning
    B. Cyanide poisoning
    C. Food poisoning
    D. Hyperthermia

93. **What immediate emergency intervention would you implement for the couple described above?**
    A. Provide them with fresh air
    B. Provide them with 100% oxygen
    C. Administer lactated Ringers
    D. Administer antiemetic

94. **Select the herb or alternative substance paired with its correct description.**
    A. Turmeric: Can be grated, boiled, and then placed on an area to relieve pain
    B. Ginger: The bark and leaves are used to treat joint pain
    C. Valerian Root: Known as nature's tranquilizer, it can be used to treat pain and insomnia
    D. Eucommia: Contains curcumin which decreases the level of two enzymes that cause inflammation

95. **Select the type of shock that is accurately paired with its cause or description.**
    A. Cardiogenic: Occurs when the ventricles of the heart are not functioning properly
    B. Anaphylactic: A systemic, multisystem response to an infection
    C. Septic: Occurs due to hemorrhage or loss of fluid from the body's circulatory system
    D. Hypovolemic: Usually occurs as the result of an allergic response to a medication

96. **What occurs during the progressive stage of shock?**
    A. Sodium ions decrease
    B. Potassium leaks from cells
    C. Blood becomes thinner
    D. Compensatory mechanisms ramp up

97. **Which of the following diseases causes blood dyscrasias that cause bleeding in the joints, significant bleeding during circumcision and easy bruising?**
    A. Idiopathic thrombocytopenic purpura
    B. Thrombotic thrombocytopenic purpura
    C. Von Willebrand's
    D. Hemophilia

98. **Disseminated intravascular coagulation:**
    A. Disrupts anticoagulation, coagulation and diaphoresis.
    B. Affects thrombosis but not bleeding.
    C. Occurs as an idiosyncratic primary condition.
    D. Is marked with excessive clotting followed by severe bleeding.

99. **Which of the following adrenal disorders is associated with adrenal hyperplasia?**
    A. Addison's syndrome
    B. Cushing's syndrome
    C. Primary aldosteronism
    D. Pheochromocytoma

100. As you are caring for a patient with type 2 diabetes, the patient expresses concerns about the acute complications of diabetes. What should you teach this patient about?
    A. The role of good blood glucose control in terms of preventing hyperglycemic
    B. The role of good blood glucose control in terms of preventing neuropathy and nephropathy
    C. The role of regular exercise in terms of preventing peripheral neuropathy
    D. The role of regular exercise in terms of preventing diabetic retinopathy

101. Illnesses and increased stress often leads to which complication of diabetes?
    A. Hyperglycemia
    B. Hypoglycemia
    C. Nephropathy
    D. Gastroparesis

102. Hyperglycemia, or high blood glucose, is defined as a fasting (8hour) blood glucose level that is more than:
    A. 160 mg/dL.
    B. 170 mg/dL.
    C. 180 mg/dL.
    D. 190 mg/dL.

103. What are the most commonly occurring pathogens that are associated with sepsis during pregnancy and the postpartum period?
    A. Yersinia pestis and Variola
    B. Yersinia pestis and Pseudomonas
    C. Variola and group A Escherichia coli
    D. Pseudomonas and Group A Escherichia coli

104. **Select the ethical term that is correctly and accurately paired with its description.**
    A. Beneficence: "Do not harm", as in the Hippocratic Oath
    B. Justice: Truthfulness and honesty
    C. Nonmaleficence: "Do not harm", as in the Hippocratic Oath
    D. Fidelity: Fairness and equality

105. **Without prior written consent, a patient's medical information:**
    A. Can only be shared with family members.
    B. Can only be shared with the patient's spouse or domestic partner.
    C. Can only be shared with those who are providing direct medical care to the patient.
    D. Cannot be shared with anyone.

106. **Which term is most appropriate to describe research-based practice?**
    A. Evidence-based practice
    B. Benchmarked practice
    C. A best practice
    D. Empirical research

107. **Which of the following medications is only available in combination with other ingredients?**
    A. Fentanyl
    B. Hydrocodone
    C. Codeine
    D. Morphine

108. **Which is used for the short-term management of moderately severe acute pain that would otherwise require narcotics?**
    A. Diflunisal
    B. Meclofenamate
    C. Mefenamic acid
    D. Ketorolac

109. **What types of patients should be screened for falls?**
    A. All patients
    B. The elderly
    C. The confused or elderly
    D. The confused elderly and mentally ill

110. **What is the single most effective way to prevent nosocomial infections in healthcare facilities?**
    A. Wearing a mask
    B. Wearing a gown
    C. Wearing a mask and gown
    D. Hand washing

111. **What is a difference between risk management and quality improvement?**
    A. Risk management aims to identify and reduce liability by eliminating risks and liabilities
    B. Risk management is proactively planning change
    C. Quality improvement is aimed at identifying problems and reporting the serious ones
    D. Quality improvement is aimed at eliminating risks for future problems

112. **Successful delegation is most dependent on:**
    A. The legal and appropriate matching of patient needs with staff competencies.
    B. The leadership and conflict resolution skills of the person who is delegating.
    C. The preferences of the patients, significant others and staff members.
    D. Specificity of the delegated assignments and follow up supervision

113. **What is the name of the process used to dig down to the real reasons why mistakes and errors have occurred?**
    A. Peer review
    B. Root cause analysis
    C. Variance tracking
    D. Benchmarking

114. Your newly diagnosed cancer patient is being discharged from the hospital. Her husband reports that he will not be able to care for her right now because he has to give his job two weeks' notice. He will be available to care for her after ten work days are over. He also expresses feeling overwhelmed with all his new responsibilities and wants to be able to take time off as a caregiver once in a while. What level of hospice care is appropriate for this caregiver at this time?

    A. Routine home care
    B. Continuous home care
    C. Respite care
    D. General inpatient care

115. Which hormones does the thyroid gland secrete?

    A. T2 and T3
    B. T3 and T4
    C. T4 and T5
    D. T5 and T6

116. Select the ASIA scale grade that is accurately paired with its characteristic deficits.

    A. Grade A: The least severe of all
    B. Grade B: The lack of motor function below the level of the injury
    C. Grade C: The lack of sensory function above the level of the injury
    D. Grade D: The most severe of all

117. The primary causative agent associated with Guillain-Barre syndrome is:

    A. Campylobacter jejuni
    B. coli
    C. HIV
    D. Legionella bacteria

118. Guillain-Barre syndrome is characterized with:

    A. Jacksonian March
    B. Tonic clonic seizures
    C. Ascending paralysis

D. Descending paralysis

119. Which of the following is the most life threatening neurological disorder?

   A. Guillain-Barre syndrome
   B. Temporal arteritis
   C. Parasympathetic neuropathy
   D. Sympathetic neuropathy

120. Legionnaire's disease is what type of infectious disease?
   A. Gastrointestinal
   B. Neurological
   C. Cardiovascular
   D. Respiratory

121. Which medication is used for both cancer pain and facial nerve pain?
   A. Phenytoin
   B. Oxcarbazepine
   C. Carbamazepine
   D. Levetiracetam

122. Corneal abrasions secondary to Bell's palsy can be best prevented with:
   A. Prednisone
   B. Moistening eye drops
   C. Methylprednisolone
   D. A humidifier

123. A three year-old pediatric patient comes to the ER and his mother states that the child has "stuffed a cooked mushroom in his ear". What complication specific to the mushroom must be considered by the nurse?

   A. An allergic nasopharyngeal response
   B. A foul smelling ear discharge
   C. Swelling of the nasal passages
   D. Swelling of the internal ear

124. The mother of a four year-old child presents at the emergency department stating that the child has "a weird cold" because their nose is running profusely but only from the left nostril. What is this child most likely affected with?

    A. A foreign body in the left nostril
    B. A foreign body in the right nostril
    C. A blunt force trauma to the left nostril
    D. A blunt force trauma to the right nostril

125. A pediatric patient presents in the emergency department with the signs of a ruptured tympanic membrane. Physical examination using an auroscope shows no presence of a foreign body. The mother of the child appears somewhat nervous and agitated. What would you most likely do?

    A. Suspect that the mother has been negligent
    B. Treat the child with antibiotic ear drops
    C. Restrain the child in a flat, supine position
    D. Suspect child abuse and report it accordingly

126. Which is a possible cause of a ruptured tympanic membrane?

    A. Influenza
    B. Sky diving
    C. Swimming in a pool
    D. Rapid running

127. Which health care professional is most likely able to diagnose problems with the temporomandibular joint?

    A. A nurse
    B. An occupational therapist
    C. A dentist
    D. A physical therapist

128. The treatment of a temporomandibular joint dislocation includes the manual pushing of the:

    A. Mandible downwards and backwards
    B. Mandible upwards and backwards
    C. Maxilla downwards and backwards
    D. Maxilla upwards and backwards

129. Which of the following is the most sight-threatening ocular condition?
   A. Corneal abrasion
   B. Corneal laceration
   C. Retinal detachment
   D. Iritis

130. What disorder can cause facial muscles to abnormally contract?

   A. Damage to the eighth cranial nerve
   B. Hypocalcemia
   C. Damage to the tenth cranial nerve
   D. Hypercalcemia

131. The ASIA scale is a scoring scale for what type of disorder or disease?
   A. Cerebrovascular accidents
   B. Blast injuries
   C. Gastrointestinal cancers
   D. Spinal cord injuries

132. Select the type of shunt that is accurately paired with its description.
   A. Ventriculo-Peritoneal Shunts: Move fluid from abdominal ascites
   B. Ventriculo-Pleural Shunts: Move fluid into the heart
   C. Ventriculo-Atrial Shunts: Move fluid to the right atrium of the heart
   D. Ventriculo-Atrial Shunts: Move fluid to the left atrium of the heart

133. The diagnosis of temporal arteritis is done with:
   A. Biopsy
   B. CT scan
   C. MRI
   D. Blood for Epstein Barr

134. **Which is the most serious and most life-threatening complication of pregnancy?**
    A. Hyperemesis gravidarum
    B. Vena cava syndrome
    C. Eclampsia
    D. Aortocaval compression

135. **A pregnant woman comes to the ER and collapses. In what position is this pregnant woman placed for CPR?**
    A. On the right side and angled backward at a 30 degree angle
    B. On the left side and angled backward at a 30 degree angle
    C. On the right side and angled forward at a 45 degree angle
    D. On the left side and angled forward at a 45 degree angle

136. **What is the most severe complication of rubella exposure among pregnant women?**

    A. Maternal collapse
    B. Maternal eclampsia
    C. Fetal collapse
    D. Fetal cerebral palsy

137. **You are discharging a pregnant woman with endometritis from the emergency department. What should be included in this patient's discharge instructions?**

    A. The nee to monitor for dependent edema
    B. The need to monitor blood pressure twice a day
    C. The need to continue the anti-hypertensives as ordered
    D. The need to continue the antibiotics as ordered

138. **Which statement about exophthalmos is accurate?**
    A. Exophthalmos occurs after an ocular blast injury.
    B. Exophthalmos primarily occurs with globe rupture.
    C. Exophthalmos is protruding eyeballs.
    D. Exophthalmos is a genetic disorder.

139. Which of the following is the highest priority need for the pregnant woman with pyelonephritis?

    A. Pain
    B. Insomnia
    C. Altered urinary elimination
    D. Urinary urgency

140. A pregnant woman comes to the ER with obvious signs of facial trauma and bruising. Her husband appears agitated and hostile. What is the first thing that you would do?

    A. Call the police because you suspect abuse
    B. Apply ice to the woman's face to relieve swelling
    C. Separate the couple to collect assessment data
    D. Notify your supervisor about spousal abuse

141. As you are assessing the pregnant woman described above, she complains of abdominal cramping. The gynecologist examines the patient and determines that the woman is at 18 weeks of gestation, has dilated 3cm and is 40% effaced. What is the nurse's immediate, priority action?

    A. Place the patient in the left lateral Sim's position
    B. Prepare for preterm labor secondary to trauma
    C. Instruct the mother to remain in bed at home for 2 days
    D. Report the obvious spousal abuse

142. Which of the following is a sign of severe preeclampsia?

    A. The Harlequin sign
    B. A positive Babinski sign
    C. Microangiopathic hemolytic anemia
    D. Nuchal rigidity and back arching

143. Which patient is at greatest risk for hyperparathyroidism?
    A. A 32 year old male with cancer of the testes
    B. A 72 year old male with cancer of the prostate
    C. A 32 year old female with stage 1 breast cancer
    D. A 72 year old female in good health

144. Your patient is discharged home with a prescription for ticlopidine. What information about this medication should you educate this patient about?
    A. The oral bid dosage of 250 mg on an empty stomach
    B. The oral bid dosage of 500 mg on an empty stomach
    C. The oral bid dosage of 250 mg with food
    D. The oral bid dosage of 500 mg with food

145. Which is the most serious life-threatening complication associated with ticlopidine?
    A. Deep vein thrombosis
    B. Nausea and vomiting
    C. Thrombotic thrombocytopenic purpura
    D. Pernicious anemia

146. Which anatomical structure should you be able to normally palpate during a physical assessment?
    A. The thyroid gland
    B. The liver
    C. The gallbladder
    D. The parathyroid gland

147. A patient with a known aldosterone deficiency has presented in the emergency department. You have taken his vital signs and his pulse is weak; the rate is 47 beats per minute. Which disorder would you suspect?
    A. Hypercalcemia
    B. Hyponatremia
    C. Hyperkalemia
    D. Hypokalemia

148. What emergency treatment would be indicated for the aldosterone deficiency patient described above?
    A. Intravenous fluids and a loop diuretic
    B. Intravenous fluids and potassium replacement
    C. Medications to reverse the alkalosis
    D. The administration of cation exchange resins

149. Which is the primary cause and risk factor associated with pheochromocytoma?
  A. Genetics
  B. Excessive exposure to ultraviolet light
  C. An adrenal gland tumor
  D. Color blindness

150. What is the most serious complication of hypothyroidism?
  A. Myxedema
  B. Thyroid storm
  C. Systemic edema
  D. Negentropy

151. After a thorough assessment of the emergency department patient, the patient is diagnosed with temporal arteritis. What should you include in the discharge teaching for this patient?
  A. The need to avoid milk and other dietary sources of calcium
  B. The need to avoid all forms of aspirin regardless of dosage
  C. The side effects of methotrexate
  D. The side effects of ACE inhibitors

152. Which statement about shunt malfunction is accurate?
  A. Shunt malfunctions are defined as an obstruction of the shunt.
  B. Shunt malfunctions are defined as the migration of the shunt.
  C. Shunt malfunctions can result in over draining.
  D. Under draining can be characterized with hydrocephalus.

153. Select the sign or symptom that is accurately paired with a possible medical complication.
  A. Over draining shunts are characterized with increased intracranial pressure.
  B. Infection is the most commonly occurring complication associated with shunts.
  C. Under draining shunts are characterized with slit ventricle syndrome
  D. Papilledema is the most commonly occurring complication associated with shunts.

154. **The primary distinguishing factor that differentiates transient ischemic attacks from cerebrovascular accident is the fact that transient ischemic attacks:**
    A. Do not affect motor function like cerebrovascular accidents do.
    B. Do not affect sensory function like cerebrovascular accidents do.
    C. Can be prevented with carotid angioplasty unlike cerebrovascular accidents.
    D. Last only a few minutes with effects unlike cerebrovascular accidents.

155. **As you are discharging a patient who has just experienced a transient ischemic attack, what would you include in this patient's discharge education?**
    A. Strict bed rest for at least 4 days
    B. A diet rich in vitamin K
    C. The side effects of ticlopidine
    D. The side effects of acetylcholinesterase inhibitors

156. **You are planning on discharging a patient from the emergency department. One of the patient goals for this patient was to attain a normal calcium balance. Which laboratory data indicates the fulfilment of this goal?**
    A. A serum calcium level of 7.5 mg/dL
    B. A serum calcium level of 8.0 mg/dL
    C. A serum calcium level of 9.0 mg/dL
    D. A serum calcium level of 10.5 mg/dL

157. **What is the ultimate goal of critical incident debriefings?**
    A. Peer support and stress management
    B. Performance improvement
    C. Benchmarking
    D. Quality control and improvement

158. **What treatment would you anticipate for a patient who has been diagnosed with an Achilles tendon rupture?**
    A. Surgical shortening of the tendon
    B. Surgical release of the tendon
    C. The application of heat
    D. The administration of a NSAID

159. **Select the type of blast injury that is correctly and accurately paired with its causal factor.**
   A. Primary blast injuries: Toxic blast injury
   B. Secondary blast injuries: Pressure on internal organs
   C. Tertiary blast injuries: Blunt force trauma
   D. Miscellaneous blast injuries: Soft tissue damage

160. **Which statement about strains and sprains is accurate?**
   A. The treatment of both is essentially the same.
   B. A sprain occurs most often as the result of overuse.
   C. A strain is often results from abnormal twisting.
   D. Strains and sprains can lead to compartment syndrome.

161. **Which is the greatest physiological danger associated with paint ball games?**
   A. A strain
   B. A sprain
   C. A laceration
   D. Lens damage

162. **An example of a psychological situational crisis that young parents are often affected with is:**
   A. The loss of a loved one
   B. Sudden infant death
   C. The loss of a spouse
   D. The loss of personal possessions

163. **Which patient is at greatest risk of aspiration pneumonia?**
   A. Patients who are taking long term NSAIDS
   B. A patient with a PICC line
   C. A patient with a PEG tube
   D. A patient with hypermotility

164. **Lou Gehrig's disease is:**
   A. A neurological disorder called amyotrophic lateral sclerosis
   B. A respiratory disorder called amyotrophic lateral sclerosis
   C. A musculoskeletal disorder called amyotrophic lateral sclerosis
   D. An endocrine disorder called amyotrophic lateral sclerosis

165. Which triage color is accurately paired with the level of care needed and/or the nature of the injury?

    A. Green: Life threatening injuries in need of immediate treatment

    B. Yellow: Minor injuries that require little treatment

    C. Black: Death is expected

    D. Red: Death is expected

Answer Key

1.	A	35.	C	69.	B
2.	D	36.	C	70.	D
3.	A	37.	B	71.	C
4.	A	38.	B	72.	B
5.	D	39.	B	73.	C
6.	A	40.	C	74.	A
7.	D	41.	C	75.	C
8.	A	42.	C	76.	B
9.	B	43.	C	77.	A
10.	D	44.	A	78.	A
11.	A	45.	C	79.	D
12.	B	46.	D	80.	B
13.	D	47.	A	81.	A
14.	B	48.	B	82.	C
15.	A	49.	D	83.	A
16.	B	50.	B	84.	A
17.	B	51.	C	85.	B
18.	A	52.	B	86.	D
19.	A	53.	D	87.	A
20.	C	54.	A	88.	D
21.	D	55.	C	89.	D
22.	C	56.	A	90.	A
23.	D	57.	B	91.	C
24.	A	58.	C	92.	A
25.	A	59.	A	93.	B
26.	C	60.	A	94.	C
27.	D	61.	C	95.	A
28.	A	62.	D	96.	B
29.	C	63.	C	97.	D
30.	D	64.	A	98.	D
31.	B	65.	C	99.	C
32.	A	66.	B	100.	A
33.	D	67.	B	101.	A
34.	A	68.	C	102.	C

103. D	124. A	145. C
104. C	125. D	146. A
105. C	126. B	147. C
106. A	127. C	148. D
107. B	128. A	149. C
108. D	129. C	150. A
109. A	130. B	151. C
110. D	131. D	152. C
111. A	132. C	153. B
112. A	133. A	154. D
113. B	134. C	155. D
114. C	135. B	156. C
115. B	136. D	157. A
116. B	137. D	158. D
117. A	138. C	159. C
118. C	139. A	160. A
119. A	140. C	161. D
120. D	141. B	162. B
121. C	142. C	163. C
122. B	143. D	164. A
123. D	144. C	165. C

Made in the USA
Middletown, DE
28 November 2015